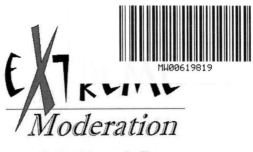

Moderation

A Handbook For Fitness Professionals

By: Kip Russo and Robb Kelly

Become an Expert in:

- ✓ **Nutrition**
- ✓ **Exercise**
- ✓ **Supplements**
- ✓ **Anti-Oxidants**
- ✓ **Hormone Modulation**

Disclaimer

Published by Ponderosa Publishers Renton, WA

Copyright © 2006 by Kip Russo and Robb Kelly
ISBN: **1-59971-526-0**

Additional copies can be ordered by contacting the publisher directly:
19910 118th Ave SE
Renton, WA 98058

email: Ponderosa@Q45.net   phone:206-427-0898

Printed in the United States of America.

| Table of Contents | Page Number |

Introduction to: *"The Plan"*

Chapter One

This is a no-nonsense plan specifically designed to allow you to finally get in the kind of physical shape you have dreamed about. It does not have all the boring filler stuff necessary to fill the chapters of a book. This is not intended to supply entertainment. Our premise is to tell it like it is, with enough pertinent information to allow you to design and obtain the body you have dreamed about. It is possible now, and it can and will become a reality if you take it to heart. Don't skip anything and if you don't completely understand every section, go back and read it again. This is an educational, lifestyle change, (a behavior change), which will result in a total body change.

Our program is not the traditional, caloric deprivation program that is tailored to allow you to prevail temporarily, or rely on us for continued support, food or supplements. We don't tell you how many points, calories, good carbohydrates, low fat, high protein, etc., to eat. Those types of plans are generally gimmickry or difficult to adhere to. We don't require follow-up sessions. We don't require you to buy our food. We approach your nutritional intake as having been a life long problem that you have been unable to solve by yourself, and it has finally manifested itself to a point where it is no longer tolerable. That is why none of the previous diets you have tried have worked. Don't feel bad because, in the long term, those programs don't work for anyone else either. We address the problem. Most programs are a temporary fix that work for a few weeks, then you can't continue them for a variety of reasons.

Hence, we'll take the approach that you want to permanently change your health and appearance and are willing to do whatever it takes to finally make it a reality, "A PERMANENT LIFESTYLE CHANGE". Such a major undertaking can't be done with a simple plan. It requires a lot more. And, for this program to work, which it will, you need to agree to the following: To successfully be on the path of a life long health and fitness plan. This is what you have long dreamed about and finally deserve. When you are willing to humble yourself and sacrifice, you can learn to achieve the ultimate goal of longevity. After all, we all have heard the story about the person who said, "My grandfather smoked cigarettes every day and lived to be 95 years old", or the person who says, "My grandparents drank whiskey every day and lived to be 95 years old". However, none of us can say, "My grandfather was 350 pounds and lived to be 95 years old", because he didn't. He's dead! He died an average of 13 years earlier than his non-obese counterpart.

In today's' politically correct environment, your doctor, your friends, and your family won't "tell it like it is" for fear of being criticized as being cruel or heartless. However, the reality is, regardless of how you look or don't look, current statistics indicate that if you are obese, you are probably going to die 13 years earlier than you would if you were fit. This assumption is presuming you are over 30% body fat. If you are not, and you are reading this, you probably would have been, had you not decided to do something. Congratulations!

We are interested in your body and the length and quality of your life, not what may or may not make you feel better about yourself. As you help yourself get fit, feeling better about yourself is an automatic byproduct of the ongoing process, its just not our focus here.

Actually, there are reasons other than simply overeating. Granted, overeating is the prime reason most people are fat. Overeating does need to be reeled-in to the reasonable constraints of what our body needs. But what does it need? These statements about "being fat is not your fault" are nonsense. Accountability and truthful awareness is crucial for success.

Most "educated" fitness and weight loss experts unanimously agree that Obesity (over 30% Body Fat in most cases) is a result of the following five factors in order of importance:

1. **Obsessive/Compulsive behavior**. This, if agreed to by you as being a partial cause, can be remedied by sound practices of Behavior Modification. Habit breaking is required, and is a part of this program. Countless numbers of previous clients, who felt they were destined to live in huge bodies, have made remarkable progress. However, the first step is being honest with yourself, agreeing that you have a compulsive eating problem, and then committing to a new lifestyle. An "eating disorder" is usually referred to as being the skinny person who purges, but even more than that it is the very overweight person who simply can not control themselves around food. If you think that you don't eat too much, and you can cut back any time, go surf the web for another gimmick plan. This program is not for you.

2. **Lack of education**. How many times have we heard that "I know all I need to do is push back from the table to lose weight"? That can't be farther from the truth. In simply pushing away from the table, you often deprive your body from the essential building blocks it needs to be strong and fit, and you create a carbohydrate craving that can only be satisfied by continued eating. This program is focused on making you an expert on nutrition. Lack of nutritional knowledge is another reason we CHOOSE to eat the wrong foods, if you can call them foods. Not knowing the ramifications of what food "CAN DO TO YOU" instead of what food "CAN DO FOR YOU" generally ends up with our making the choice to *eat what makes us happy*. However, by the end of this program, you will be nutritionally educated to the point where you will understand all of the fad diets, how they work, why they won't work for you, and best of all, WHAT WILL WORK FOR YOU!

3. **Exercise**. Although 85% of fitness is nutrition, exercise is the other vital 15%. This program offers guidelines for performance

8

that can only be reached by having a properly designed exercise program that is specific to you. We will point you in the right direction. We'll also give you guidelines on how to hire an educated, informed, personal trainer who wants you to reach the same realistic goals you want to reach for yourself.

4. **Hormones**. If you are within 80% of the population, and are a female over 40 or a male over 50, hormones are a factor. Don't you ever wonder why you used to be able to eat more and not exercise, yet you were fitter and thinner than you are now? Or, why does one man who eats 5,000 calories a day grow to 350 pounds, and another man who eats the same amount of calories per day, grows to 600 pounds? What happens to men's bellies after 50, and why do their arms seem to shrink? Women, what happens to them after 40? They exercise, think they are eating right, yet can't seem to stop gaining weight? They add more and more aerobics to their exercise plan yet continue to gain. At the end of this program, you will understand exactly what part hormones play in your body. You will know exactly where your hormone levels should be, and how to get them to the point where they maximize your energy, fat loss and muscular gain. Yep! You are going to understand it all. On the other hand, if you are one of the unfortunate 5% of the population, hormones are the primary reason you have been fat for most, if not all of your life. That can be fixed as well.

5. **Genetics**. It is a mitigating factor in the caloric assimilation process, but probably not the reason you are fat.

- You can not burn or utilize more food than you have the ability to eat, unless you are a world class athlete, and I mean "world class".

- Most overweight people eat more food than their body needs to function, repair itself, and exist in a healthy, energetic manner.

- If you eat or consume fewer calories than your body burns, you will **ALWAYS LOSE WEIGHT**. *There are no exceptions to this rule unless your hormones are way out of balance, or unless you are on specific medication that inhibits weight loss.*

- If you do not consume enough protein to satisfy the demand you are putting on your muscles, you will not gain the level of muscularity that you are already demanding your muscles to attain through your current fitness program. You need to either increase your protein intake to the amount your body requires, or cut your exercise program back. There is no point in wasting your time, is there?

- If you do not eat before and after a strenuous workout, you will lose muscle mass.

- To determine how many calories your body requires to function per day, which will allow you to determine how many calories you need to subtract to lose FAT, you must know your RMR (Resting Metabolic Rate). If you have been Hydrostatically Tested by Body Fat Test, your RMR is at the bottom of the third page of your report. If you have not been tested by us, you need to be tested to move forward in this process. Go to the "nutritional" link on the Body Fat Test website that shows the locations where Body Fat Test is going to be testing. Contact the facility closest to you and make an appointment. Once you have been tested, and have your Resting Metabolic Rate in hand, read on. Without your RMR, the rest of this program will not work for you.

- Now that you know your RMR, you need to add the number of additional calories that you burn doing various activities. This number is on the last page of your report. The combination of these two numbers will yield the total number of calories per day that you expend, or the total number of calories per day that you need to maintain your current weight. Therefore, to maintain your weight, you need to consume that amount of calories.

- One pound of fat contains 3,500 calories. 3,500 calories divided by 7 days in a week, is 500 calories per day that you need to subtract from your total daily caloric requirement, to lose one pound of fat per week. You may be tempted to double the 500 per day caloric reduction so you can lose 2 pounds per week. However, most research indicates that if you lose more than 1.5 pounds of body weight per week, you will lose lean mass as well as fat. We need all the lean mass that we can get. So, take it slow. This formula is simple math.

- Here is the rub. We presume all your hormones are in balance. As an example, the formula used to determine your RMR assumes you fall right in the middle of the normal thyroid range, which is between .35 and 5.5. The thyroid is the gland that drives our metabolism. The normal range is a HUGE range. However, most in the medical profession considers you "normal" if you fall anywhere within that range. If you are lower, your RMR will be higher. If you are higher, your RMR will be lower. Strange, but a lower thyroid number means your metabolism is faster than were you normal. If you have a concern about your hormones, get all of your levels tested. If you are male, get your thyroid, T3 and T4, plus testosterone levels checked. If you are female, add estrogen and progesterone to the list of tests you will need. Once you get the tests back (be sure and ask the doctor to give you a copy, you can get educated as to your numbers and where you fall. If you fall on either side of the "right in the middle" normal range, you will have to "guesstimate" how that may affect your RMR. Later, we will talk about Hormone Modulation, and you will then better understand how the whole thing comes together. If you think you fall within the category of needing hormone balancing, that section deals a lot more with the specific blood tests necessary for male and female hormone modulation.

- Muscle can not turn to fat and vice versa. However, muscle can atrophy and automatically adjust to a reduced load you put on them while you are overeating and getting fatter. Muscle can also expand and become denser if you increase the load that you put on them, while your fat is being metabolized as a result of diminished caloric intake, and metabolism increases when you add lean mass. You pick, either way is your choice, but fat does not magically change into the muscle, and neither does atrophied muscle magically change its molecular structure into fat.

- Does exercise solve the obesity problem? It greatly helps, but think about this. If you consume 6 ounces of chocolate cake that contains approximately 1,050 calories. With a typical RMR of around 1,500 and if you walk at a moderate pace (3.0 miles per hour), you will burn 228 calories per hour. Therefore, you will have to walk 4.6 hours, or 13.8 miles to burn up that slice of cake. Hello!!! <u>Exercise is not the solution to weight loss</u>. It is a major factor, but not the solution. Doesn't it make more sense to forgo the 4.6 hours of walking the 13.8 miles, and just don't eat the darn piece of cake in the first place (or whatever your obsessive choice may be). Are you catching on???? Restraint, education, and proper choices are the answer. *God designed us to eat for fuel and the replenishment of vitamins, minerals and protein.* That is why the excess stuff you are consuming is stored all over your body. Yet, since there will probably never be a major famine in your lifetime (which the reason we store excess calories), the storage tanks keep getting larger and larger. Our goal is to reverse the process.

More to learn

Without knowledge, the program will not work for you. So, take notes and understand.

- **One gram of fat contains 9 calories**. Fat is more dense in calories than any of its counterparts, carbohydrates, or protein. Fat is primarily stored fuel. It is almost always stored and not immediately used by the body because the body prefers to fuel itself off of carbohydrates. Fat can only be accessed for use as fuel, if the carbohydrate intake is lower than what is needed to fuel the body at that particular time. Then, and only then, is the fat accessed and used as fuel. As you know, this condition (very few carbohydrates recently ingested) seldom exists in today's culture. Fat has little value, other than the few essential fatty acids that our body needs to make hormones, cushion vital body organs, and it is stored as a long term fuel.

- **One gram of a carbohydrate contains 4 calories.** Carbohydrates are generally all foods that are not from an animal or comprised of fat. Carbohydrates range from simple table sugar, a slice of bread, a candy bar, to broccoli, carrots, fruit, etc. Carbohydrates vary greatly in their caloric content. You will need to select the low calorie, color rich vegetables as they contain the most vitamins, minerals, and anti-oxidants. Later,we will discuss the *glycemic index* that you need to consider when choosing carbohydrates. Carbohydrates are primarily used as instantaneous fuel once they are converted by the liver to glucose. Excess carbohydrates are also secondarily stored for use as long term fuel in the form of glycogen, which is stored in the muscles and liver. Even beyond that carbohydrates that are too excessive to be stored as glycogen, once the storage stores are full, are converted to triglycerides, which are stored as fat. Carbohydrates are the body's primary source of vitamins and minerals. All of the organs in the body including the muscles receive fuel from glucose. Glucose is the basic chemical that ALL carbohydrates are broken down into. When there is a low glucose level in the blood, the body still needs fuel, so it turns to stored fat. If your carbohydrate intake is high, you will not burn fat because carbohydrate fuel (glucose) will be used instead. On the other hand, the brain is the only organ in the body that can not use fat for fuel. If there is a low blood glucose level, the brain will instruct your body to metabolize its fat so that the body can fuel itself off of the fat and the resulting ketones. This allows the last bit of glucose to be set aside for use by the brain. In an effort to avoid getting too technical, let's just say that it is impossible to add lean muscle mass while on a caloric restricted diet. To gain lean mass, your body needs to be in a positive energy state, or high in calories. That means, your body needs all the calories necessary to function at the current activity level, plus enough additional calories needed to add lean mass. Therefore, it is impossible to have it both ways (lose fat while gaining muscle). So, our program is designed to help you retain as much muscle mass as possible while reducing the stored fat. You should focus on building lean mass once you are nearer your fat reduction goal.

- **One gram of protein contains 4 calories.** Protein, which is a combination of specific amino acids, is the only food which is used to repair, replace, and replenish, your muscle and organ tissue. Protein is very seldom used as fuel, but excess protein also, can be converted to fat and glucose. Protein is the primary building block of our Life. Hence, our nutritional intake should be based around an adequate protein intake which is dictated by our lean mass and activity level. Of the many amino acids that comprise protein, some are essential to be effective and others are not. As an example, legumes have certain amino acids, but do not comprise all of the essential 9 amino acids. To properly replenish your muscles and organs, you need 21 amino acids in combination. Amino acids are the foundation of all life. Of the 21 amino acids, nine of them, known as the essential amino acids, cannot be synthesized by the human body and must be supplied by the diet. Without these essential amino acids constantly entering the body, the rates of new protein formation will slow down, and in the extreme case, stop altogether. You can see why having adequate levels of protein on a daily basis is critical. You must constantly provide the foundation for new protein formation, and it must be high-quality, digestible protein. Therefore, the legumes will not do the job by themselves. Legumes are an incomplete protein. Although they do contain some of the essential 9 amino acids, they don't contain all 9. Rice has the necessary "essential" amino acids that are lacking in the beans. On the other hand rice, by itself is an incomplete protein as well. Therefore, beans and rice separately are not complete proteins because they do not contain all of the essential amino acids. Combined, beans and rice contain all of the essential amino acids required by the body. They are considered to be a "complete protein" as do all meat and dairy products, independently, as well as the vegetable "soy". Your Nutritional plan will be structured around obtaining the proper amount of protein based on your lean mass retention requirements and your exercise level. The balance of your daily caloric intake will come from a balance of carbohydrates and fat. If you are, and intend to remain a couch potato with little or no exercise, protein is of little consequence because you are not putting a muscular demand on your body. However, if you follow our plan to make your body a fat burning, strong, lean machine, you will need adequate protein at each meal and snack to maximize the facilitation of this result. Protein is not used as fuel when caloric supply is adequate. The body's primary fuel choices are carbohydrates and fats. If carbohydrates are not adequate, protein can be converted to fat and glucose via gluconeogenesis. The best sources of protein are eggs, milk, and meat. Certain vegetable proteins can be eaten together or with animal proteins to compliment proteins for proper amino-acid ratios. Some of these vegetables are beans. Soybeans are a complete protein all by themselves. Other complimentary proteins are: grains, kidney beans, white beans, lima beans, lentils, chick peas, green peas, black-eyed peas, bread, pasta, rice, bulgur, corn, almonds, sesame seed, and peanuts. Keep in mind, however, that many protein containing vegetables are also high in carbohydrates, and some are even high in fat, such as avocados. Therefore, the caloric content of a protein obtained from a combination of two or more carbohydrates may be much higher in calories than the same quantity of protein obtained from a dairy or meat source.

- **One gram of fiber contains 0 calories.** Fiber is primarily non-digestible and therefore has no calories. Fiber can attach itself to fat and keep the fat from being digested in the small intestine. The huge benefit of fiber is its ability to keep your bowels regular. Without regularity, you may accumulate in excess of 25 pounds of undigested feces which adheres to the intestinal walls and will ultimately make you sick. This putrid waste can add to the potential of colon cancer as well as keeping the digestive tract from being as efficient as it was designed to be. You should get most of your fiber from breakfast. Choose your first meal of the day with fiber in mind. Adults should have a minimum of 30 grams of fiber in their daily intake from all meals and snacks. With some cereals, you can get as much as 16 grams of fiber from that one meal. You can determine if you are getting enough fiber by the quality and number of bowel movements that you have daily. The goal should be two bowel movements daily. One is okay, but two is optimal.

"When I am on the go, I eat a bowl of "Go Lean" cereal. When I am at home, I cook my special concoction of oatmeal and other grains. I will supply the recipe later –Kip".

- If you have a low glucose blood level, resulting from diminished carbohydrate intake, you will lose fat. This sounds contradictory, because earlier we said "eat more carbohydrates". However, we mean high quality, low glycemic load carbohydrates, because they are generally lower in calories. Low caloric carbohydrates aid in the access of stored fat. High caloric carbohydrates, such as sugar, candy, rice, potatoes, will result in the storage of additional fat, not the metabolization of already stored fat.

- Insulin is the hormone that reduces the amount of sugar (glucose) that is free in the blood stream. The brain needs to operate within a certain envelope of blood sugar level. If the blood sugar gets too high as a result of being uncontrolled by insulin (Diabetes), you can go into shock. If your blood sugar gets too low as a result of too little carbohydrate intake, you will feel lethargic. When the glucose level is over abundant, the pancreas secretes insulin. Insulin decreases the level of glucose by converting the excess glucose into glycogen (glucose in a concentrated storage form), which is stored in the liver and muscles for future use.

- If the glucose level is too low, the pancreas secretes glucagon. Glucagon is the opposite of insulin. Glucagon is the chemical that increases the amount of glucose in the blood stream by freeing glycogen (concentrated glucose stored in the liver). Although, glycogen is stored in the muscle and in the liver, glycogen can only be freed from the liver by glucagon, which allows the glycogen to be metered back in the blood stream for use as fuel. The glycogen in the muscle is specifically restricted for use by the muscle as needed. However, when in a "fight or flight" situation, high amounts of glycogen is released from the muscles as a result of the hormone adrenalin, which is secreted by the pituitary gland. Adrenalin causes the increased volume release of fuel directly into the muscle, which is why we have such intensified strength and speed when we are frightened or startled.

- Vitamins and Minerals are primarily obtained <u>in their natural form</u> from carbohydrates that were once grown, i.e. vegetables and fruit. Some minerals do come from meat but mostly from carbohydrates.

Jack LaLane once said, "I eat for fuel and rejuvenation. That is the way God designed us". If that be the case, why else should we eat? Because you are hungry, bored, lonely, angry, anxious, etc.? NO! We are killing ourselves prematurely, one mouthful at a time, and you feel awful most of the time. You are now being offered all of the information necessary that will extend your life by an average of 13 years, during which time, you will feel more energetic, look better, and have a sense of well being that you haven't experienced in years.

Serious Fat Loss Program

Congratulations! If you have made it this far, you are on your way to one of the best decisions of your life. The commitment to learn more about healthy eating habits is the first step toward making a healthy, positive change in your life. This knowledge will also free you from all the future fad diets that most frustrated/overweight people will succumb to and fail. We will show you how to get started and how to succeed on a customized weight management program that will be a life change for you.

Your program will be created exclusively for you, by you, based on your metabolic rate, lifestyle and exercise plan. This program is not just specific to weight loss. You will need to strive to maintain and increase muscular mass and improve your overall physical condition while on the path to reach your optimum weight goal.

First, let's see if you have been paying attention. To understand how the process works, you need to have the incremental facts committed to your memory.

Test number one:

1. *How many calories in one gram of fat?*
2. *How many calories in one gram of carbohydrates?*
3. *How many calories in one gram of protein?*
4. *How many calories in one gram of fiber?*
5. *What are carbohydrates used for by the body?*
6. *What are fats used for by the body?*
7. *What is protein used for by the body?*
8. *What is fiber used for by the body?*
9. *What is the primary purpose of insulin?*
10. *What is your RMR?*
11. *What is the rule to which there are "**No Exceptions**"?*
12. *How many calories does one pound of fat contain?*
13. *How many calories will you need to subtract from your total caloric requirements to lose one and a half pounds per week?*

I don't know how you did, but if you had trouble with any of the questions, you should go back and re-read each section that addresses the areas where you are weak.

What is the Bottom Line?

We realize that you have tried everything without success: low fat, high protein, low carbohydrate, cabbage diet, grapefruit diet, etc. Now that you have found this program, it is absolutely essential that you adapt the attitude that this program is going to work for you and you are willing to devote 3 months to make it work.

If you do so, it will work, and it will establish new habits to enable the new lifestyle to be permanent.

Without this commitment, you ARE going to be <u>fat for the rest of your life</u>.

Behavior Modification

B.F. Skinner, a noted psychologist and behavior modification expert, indicates that if you continue a new behavior consistently for a period of 27 to 30 days, it can become a new habit. New habits are what we are trying to create in our new way of eating. It also takes 27 to 30 days of consistent change to break a bad habit.

Before we can try to change a behavior, we must first acknowledge that we would like to change a certain behavior. This applies to everything we do, from eating too much ice cream to speeding on the highway. *For some people, deciding to make a change is the most difficult step in the process of change.* <u>A change means a change</u>. You can't meter it in gradually. You must make the change and cut old ties completely. Since you are this far in your reading in hopes that we could motivate you to finally make a change in your current eating habits and lifestyle, please allow us to help you make the commitment to finally get into the kind of shape you have dreamed of being in. It is not only possible, it is probable. Make the commitment, or throw this package away and stop reading. <u>You must do it to succeed</u>.

Once you know that there is something you would like to change, the next step is gaining the knowledge of how to change. Once you have all of the ingredients -- the awareness that you need to make a change, the cognition of knowing how to change, and the emotion and drive of actually wanting to change -- you're ready to make the decision to change. Finally, the last step to successfully change a behavior is to *take action!* **This action starts when you finish this paragraph. Enough**

18

is enough. Are you not sick and tired of being sick and tired? Get off of your butt, and make a commitment to yourself. Say to yourself, over and over again, until you have a life commitment, "I WILL STOP CONTRIBUTING TO BEING A FAT PERSON".

To change one must change their thinking, believing, expectations, attitude, performance, and behavior. All of these changes will result in changing your life. Thinking and believing what you want, will promote speaking about what you want, will promote acting on want you want, and finally this action will provide results.

Remember this statement: Wish →Want→Need →Got. We hear people all the time **wish** they were in better shape but they never do anything about it. Taking it to the next level are the people who really **want** something and they are usually speaking out about it but still may not be doing anything. The final level before the goal is the **need** stage. These people are actually doing it, taking action. You don't hear them, rather you see them, taking action because they know deep down they need to have it and will stop at nothing to get it. They might even seem a little fanatical at times but maybe that is what you need to do too – get fanatical about getting fit, it's that important, don't you think?

De-Calorie Your House.

Simple restraint, no matter how good the intentions, **will not work**. So, go to the pantry, the drawers and the refrigerator. Get rid of the cookies, cakes, ice cream, salad dressing, butter, margarine, sugar, white bread, and everything that "God did not create in its natural form". If you are worried about wasting food, give it to a friend. They will love it, and be very appreciative, but get it out of your house.

Subtract add-on-fats from all of your foods, and get them out of the house. A lot of the foods we eat are naturally low in fat, for example, pasta, chicken, turkey, fruits and vegetables,--until we heap them with extras like butter, dressing, gravy and sour or whipped cream. Start your new lifestyle by using substitutes for such fatty add-ons that you used to liberally apply on everything. Some ideas are Molly McButter, Fat Free Mayonnaise, Mustard or Salsa.

If you must eat regular cheese, you can't. So, forget it. Get the cheese out of the house as well. On your cheat day, you can choose low-fat cheese. That means you can only splurge with cheese on the weekend. Do not cheat and eat cheese during the week. Cheese is one of the most common fat boosters in a Woman's diet. Most cheeses average about 66 percent of calories from fat, but some shoot well into the 80 percent range. You can generally distinguish high and low-fat varieties by their color. White cheeses like mozzarella, Swiss, Ricotta and Parmesan are lower in fat than yellow cheeses like Cheddar and American. You should eventually eliminate cheese altogether, except for that occasional special occasion, at which time we all can indulge with restraint. The one cheese you can have is cottage cheese. It's a great source of calcium and protein. Choose the 1% or even fat free kind. You might not like the taste of the fat free, but try several, many are better than others.

Convert to non-fat milk. If you drink whole milk, switching to 1% can cut your fat intake substantially: 1% milk gets 27 percent of its calories from fat, while whole milk gets 48 percent, and non-fat milk is pure nutrition with no fat from calories. Naturally, non-fat is where you need to end up since it has no fat and no calories from fat, but it may take a few weeks to make the conversion. However, be aware that you will want to pat yourself on the back when you go from whole milk to 1% milk and you may tend to rationalize that 1% is okay. It is not. Keep going and make a time commitment to be drinking only fat free milk within two weeks.

Milk is an excellent source of the needed protein. Generally milk and even soy milk has between .75 and 1 gram of protein in each ounce. So, drink up.

Buy lean meats. There's room for red meat in your new nutritional plan if you make the right choices. Best choices include cuts like London broil, eye of round steak and sirloin tip, which gets less than 40 percent of their calories from fat. However, be sure and trim off the fat before you cook it. Go for reasonable portions of 4 to 6 ounces, trim all visible fat off before cooking, and prepare it by broiling, grilling or baking. Beef, if chosen properly, has only one gram of fat more than chicken breast for the same 6 ounces, yet it has far more trace elements and minerals than does chicken.

You must cut out fried foods completely. They are not allowed, and soon you will not miss them. **No fried food whatsoever, at all! They generally have little nutritional value and are extremely high in fat.**

Eat more carbohydrates, but only complex unprocessed carbohydrates.

Remember, the outline and suggestions are very strict for the first month or so, or until you have a better understanding of calories and what your body needs. Once you are better educated about yourself and how your body reacts, you can modify the whole process to a more tailor-made program just for you. When that happens, there will be room for the occasional extravagancies.

One of the most important findings about proper nutrition is that if you replace fat with other foods, like carbohydrates, you can actually eat **more,** and at the same time, consume fewer calories which results in weight loss. This is because fat has over twice the calories per gram than carbohydrates, and fat is generally stored immediately as fat.

To prove this point, in one study, when people on a moderately high fat diet were told to maintain their weight for 20 weeks while switching to a low-fat, high-carbohydrate diet which was chosen from low glycemic index carbohydrates, they lost more than 11 percent of their flab. This was despite their best efforts to keep their weight consistent.

Because carbohydrates burn faster than any other kind of food, they keep the body's metabolism revving higher requiring more calories for fuel. Consequently, the less fat you have and the more lean mass you accumulate the more high energy food you need. However, as you will see later, carbohydrates in excess of what you need for 'FUEL' converts to and gets stored as fat (triglycerides), just like fat. So, choose wisely and only eat to "re-fuel" and "reconstruct". Don't eat for any other reason. If you are bored, take up a hobby, or go to the gym. Stay away from the refrigerator.

Carbohydrates are found in a wide variety of foods, for example: cereals, beans, fruit, and all vegetables. There are two kinds of carbohydrates, complex and simple. Simple carbohydrates are such items as table sugar, honey, desserts. They have already been refined or reduced to their simplest form. While complex carbohydrates are carbohydrates such as fruit and vegetables that have not been processes. Carbohydrates are key to maximal athletic performance. They are the most efficient fuel available to the muscles for aerobic exercise and the only fuel that can be used anaerobically. At a lower intensity exercise, muscles will burn a combination of fat and carbohydrate for fuel. But, during high intensity exercise, carbohydrates are used exclusively.

Carbohydrates are so important to muscles that they actually keep their own supply of carbohydrates stored within the muscle cell (glycogen).

In addition to eating more complex carbohydrates, we also recommend you do the following:

Focus on Fiber.
Once in the digestive tract, fiber tends to attract fat and bind with it. Because fiber is indigestible, it is quickly excreted, which helps to speed fat through the digestive tract before it has time to be absorbed into the blood and stored as flab. Most low glycemic index carbohydrate foods (the preferable ones) are naturally loaded with fiber, but any kind of processing tends to deplete them of fiber. When possible, eat foods whole, leaving fiber-rich skins on fruits like apples and choosing whole grain breads and cereals. Always try to include fiber in every meal. We want you to eventually cut-out breads from your normal meals and reserve them for the special occasions. They are empty calories (meaning high in calories with little other nutritional value) and are un-necessary. Whole wheat bread makes little difference. It is very high on the glycemic index and has little nutritional value. Whole wheat bread's primary value over white bread is its fiber content.

Watch out for sugar.
Sugar is a simple carbohydrate and will make you gain fat on its own. Also, many foods high in sugar are also high in fat. A Hershey bar, for example, gets more than half of its calories from fat. Cravings for sweets are often really fat cravings in disguise. If you want something sweet, try a piece of fresh fruit or occasionally enjoy a bowl of Frosted Mini Wheat's or Go Lean Crunch by Kashi, which is high in fiber, low in fat, and sweetened from Nutri-Sweet. When you are craving sugar, you can usually find a satisfying substitute. You just need to be creative when you are not having a craving. When you do crave the sweet, the alternative is the only thing available since you already de-calorie your house. Keep in mind that fresh fruit is high in vitamins and minerals, but also higher in calories than vegetables. So, eat fruit in moderation.

Glycemic Index of Carbohydrates

The Glycemic Index was developed in the early 1980's to look at how different foods affected the blood sugar levels in patients with diabetes. Shortly after, sports scientists investigated how foods with different GI scores affect performance. Simply put, the glycemic index is a scale that rates how fast certain foods are converted to glucose by the liver and therefore, become available as a source of energy in the blood stream. Foods with a high glycemic index rating require an insulin reaction, or secretion of insulin from the pancreas, to lower the high blood sugar level as a result of too much glucose in the blood stream. That scenario is not a good thing. Better would be the carbohydrate that is metered into the system slowly so that it can mostly be used as fuel by the body rather than converted to glycogen and finally, triglycerides, which ultimately end up as stored fat.

Rapid inducers of insulin:

Glycemic index of greater than 100%
Grain-based foods
        Puffed rice
        Corn flakes
        Puffed wheat
        Millet
        Instant rice
        Instant potato
        Microwave potato
        French bread
Simple sugars
        Maltose
        Glucose
Snacks
        Tofu ice cream
        Puffed-rice cakes

Glycemic index standard = 100%
Grain-based foods
        Grape nuts
        Whole-wheat bread
        Rolled oats
        Instant mashed potatoes
        White rice
        Brown rice
        Muesli
        Shredded wheat
Vegetables

        Carrots
        Parsnips
        Corn
Fruits
        Banana
        Raisins
        Apricots
        Apricots
        Papaya
        Mango
Snacks
        Ice cream (low fat)
        Corn chips
        Rye crisps

Moderate inducers of insulin

Glycemic index between 50 and 80%

Grain-based foods
        Spaghetti (white)
        Spaghetti (whole wheat)
        Pasta, other
        Pumpernickel bread
        All-bran cereal
Fruits
        Orange
        Orange Juice
Vegetables
        Peas
        Pinto beans
        Garbanzo beans
        Kidney beans (canned)
        Baked beans
        Navy beans
Simple Sugars
        Lactose
        Sucrose
Snacks
        Candy bar*
        Potato chips (with fat)*

Reduced insulin secretion:

Glycemic index between 30 and 50%

Grain-based foods
        Barley
        Oatmeal (slow-cooking)
        Whole-grain rye bread

Fruit
- Apple
- Apple juice
- Applesauce
- Pears
- Grapes
- Peaches

Vegetables
- Kidney beans
- Lentils
- Black-eyed peas
- Chick-peas
- Kidney beans (dried)
- Lima beans
- Tomato soup
- Peas

Dairy Products
- Ice Cream (high fat)*
- Milt (skim)
- Milk (whole)
- Yogurt

Glycemic index 30% or less

Fruits
- Cherries
- Plums
- Grapefruit

Vegetables
- Soy Beans*

Snacks
- Peanuts*

Note: Although you are attempting to reduce your fat intake because of its dense caloric structure, some fat content will retard the rate of absorption of carbohydrate into the body.

Rule of thumb: Low Glycemic Index foods are generally fruit or fiber rich vegetables, except for bananas, carrots, corn, and potatoes.

Glycemic Indexes and Glycemic Loads for Common Foods

The table below shows values of the Glycemic Index (GI) and Glycemic Load (GL) for a few common foods. GI's of 55 or below are considered low, and 70 or above are considered high. GL's of 10 or below are considered low, and 20 or above are considered high.

GI and GL for Common Foods				
Food	GI	Serving Size	Net Carbs	GL
Peanuts	14	4 oz (113g)	15	2
Bean sprouts	25	1 cup (104g)	4	1
Grapefruit	25	1/2 large (166g)	11	3
Pizza	30	2 slices (260g)	42	13
Lowfat yogurt	33	1 cup (245g)	47	16
Apples	38	1 medium (138g)	16	6
Spaghetti	42	1 cup (140g)	38	16
Carrots	47	1 large (72g)	5	2
Oranges	48	1 medium (131g)	12	6
Bananas	52	1 large (136g)	27	14
Potato chips	54	4 oz (114g)	55	30
Snickers Bar	55	1 bar (113g)	64	35
Brown rice	55	1 cup (195g)	42	23
Honey	55	1 tbsp (21g)	17	9
Oatmeal	58	1 cup (234g)	21	12
Ice cream	61	1 cup (72g)	16	10
Macaroni and cheese	64	1 serving (166g)	47	30
Raisins	64	1 small box (43g)	32	20
White rice	64	1 cup (186g)	52	33
Sugar (sucrose)	68	1 tbsp (12g)	12	8
White bread	70	1 slice (30g)	14	10
Watermelon	72	1 cup (154g)	11	8
Popcorn	72	2 cups (16g)	10	7
Baked potato	85	1 medium (173g)	33	28
Glucose	100	(50g)	50	50

Learning More

Additional information and values for Glycemic Index and Glycemic Load can be found at www.glycemicindex.com.

Determine how much protein you need daily by the following Protein Chart.

Protein is the basic building block of the body. If you deprive yourself of the proper amount of protein, you will either lose lean mass or you will not gain lean mass based on your exercise regimen. It is a simple premise. If you are exercising (which you will be) to a point where you are putting a demand on your body to add more lean mass, yet you are not consuming enough protein, the lean mass wants to grow stronger and more dense, but it can not without the required amount of protein. Therefore, if you are not going to get enough protein, you might just as well **cut back your workout**. Without giving your body adequate protein, you are wasting your time trying to build more lean mass. It will not happen. We will discuss lean mass later in the exercise section. However, understand the need for protein now, so you can build your plan properly. Keep in mind that an average serving of protein is the size of a deck of cards, i.e. chicken breast, lean hamburger patty, 5 oz steak, etc. That quantity of protein for the sake of generalization can be considered to be 20 grams.

Also, remember the milk.

There is one gram of protein for each ounce of milk, preferably non-fat milk or soy milk. Soy milk has a bit less protein than regular skim milk, but it does have trace elements and anti oxidants that milk does not have. We don't advocate replacing fat free milk with soy milk. However we do suggest you add soy to your diet, perhaps on your cereal to supplement your non-fat milk intake. If you can tolerate the taste of soy, you should try to make it a part of your regular diet.

Calculate your daily protein requirements.

1. Obtain your lean body mass. If you have had your body fat percentage hydrostatically tested, that is the most accurate method. Lean body mass is how much your body weighs void of fat.
2. Determine your activity factor. Activity factors are listed below based on your activity level.
    - [5] Sedentary (no formal sports activity or training), or light fitness training, such as walking.
    - [6] Moderate training (3 or occasionally 4 times a week) aerobic and/or weight training.
    - [7] Aerobic training five days per week or daily moderate weight training five days per week. *Most avid fitness club members fit in here!*
    - [8] Heavy daily weight training coupled with intense aerobic training or twice-a-day intense sports training.
3. Finally, to calculate your required daily amount of protein (in grams), locate the number nearest your lean body mass (in pounds) in the left column and go to the right to the column under the activity factor that represents your level of activity. The resulting number is the daily protein requirements for you in grams.

Lean Mass	Activity Level:			
lbs	5	6	7	8
90	45	72	81	90
100	50	70	80	100
110	55	77	88	110
120	60	84	96	120
130	65	91	104	130
140	70	98	112	140
150	75	105	120	150
160	80	112	128	160
170	85	119	136	170
180	90	126	144	180
190	95	133	152	190
200	100	140	160	200
210	105	147	168	210
220	110	154	176	220

Grams of protein required

*An example would be a person whose workout is 5 days a week (**level 7**) and has **150** pounds of lean mass. This person would require **120** grams of protein daily to reach the degree of muscularity that he is already demanding upon his muscle.*

Be constantly aware of your fat intake.

Fat makes us gain weight because it's stored in the body far more easily than either carbohydrates or protein. Fat is stored as fat. Fat can be used as fuel, but it is first stored as additional fat. Generally, if there is an inadequate supply of glucose (carbohydrates) the body will access that stored fat. Fat, as said earlier, contains twice the number of calories than either carbohydrates or protein of the same weight. The body burns the carbohydrate's calories as fuel almost immediately, while the more calorie-dense fat burns slower and is more likely to be left over and stored. Furthermore, it takes a lot of energy to turn carbohydrates and protein into flab--almost a quarter of carbohydrate calories are burned up in the conversion process alone. Peter D. Vash, M.D., assistant clinical professor of medicine at the University of California--Los Angeles. **"The fat you eat is the fat you wear,"** he says. All of which is compounded by the fact that American women tend to get 38 to 40 percent of their calories from fat--double what most experts recommend.

We need some fat in our diets to maintain the proper functioning of our bodies; too little fat is almost as dangerous as too much. However, hardly a person alive today is depriving themselves of anything by cutting way back on fat. Fat is a risk factor for cardiovascular disease, diabetes, high blood pressure, stroke, some types of cancer, including that of the colon, and a barrage of other illnesses which are too numerous to list. Since fats provide 9 calories of energy per gram, they are the most concentrated of the energy-producing nutrients. Our bodies need only very small amounts. Fats play an important role in building the membranes that surround our cells and in helping blood to clot. Once digested and absorbed, fats help the body absorb certain vitamins. Fat stored in the body cushions vital organs and protects us from extreme cold and heat. <u>You need fat in your diet</u>, but the right fat in the right amounts.

This is not a "low fat diet". We are simply teaching you that foods naturally containing fat are okay, but there is no need to ADD FAT to anything. In that statement, we are assuming that you trim all excess fat off of the meat you consume, and try to purchase the leanest of meats when making your selections. Since fat makes you fat, one of the most important things you can do for both weight loss and general health, is to limit the amount of fat that you eat.

By following the general guidelines above, you should be able to cut your fat content dramatically.

Chapter Three

Start with a good breakfast. Researchers theorize that breakfast-eaters tend to eat less fat and more carbohydrates than breakfast-skippers. Breakfast eaters also do less impulsive snacking and are generally less hungry all morning. In a Vanderbilt study, overweight breakfast-skippers who started eating breakfast lost an average of 17 pounds in 12 weeks. What's more, breakfast-eaters were better able to maintain their weight loss than breakfast-skippers.

Always have your mid-morning snack. The snack not only fills you so that you will have a more conservative lunch, it stimulates the metabolism which aids in the fuel burning process. Remember that it takes calories just to process the food that you have eaten. In some cases, like a hard boiled egg, you can burn almost as many calories digesting the egg, than the egg actually contains. We call that process a negative food or a "catabolic food".

Lunch, Snack, Dinner. Start off with the sample suggestion illustrated later, and stick to it. The frequency of consumption, although seemingly excessive, has a purpose. You will keep your metabolism revving and keep total daily calories down. This always results in your not being hungry.

Kip's breakfast cereal concoction
Make a bag of cereal from Wild Oats, Vitamin Cottage, Whole Foods, etc., starting with large rolled oats. You will need to keep the ingredients separate when you buy them, but combine them in a large bowl at home, then re-bag. Add four or five other grains to it so the total amount is about 80% oats. It adds a broad spectrum of micro nutrients if you add some 7 grain cereal form the bulk bin as well. Add about one teaspoon of bran to each cup of the final mixture. You can add a small amount of raw sesame seeds too. You should also add raisins or crainsens to taste during the cooking process.

This is your initial shopping list necessary to start your program.

- One box of protein bars (Costco)
- One container of Protein Powder (Costco)
- Yoplait yogurt
- Apples
- Brown Rice
- Box of Go Lean Cereal by Kashi for the days you don't cook cereal
- Carrots
- Celery
- Boneless Skinless Chicken Breast
- Eggs
- Fish, skinless. Any kind (frozen)
- Canned Solid White Albacore Tuna packed in water
- Vegetable medley from Costco (carrots, broccoli, cauliflower)
- Mustard
- Non Fat Mayonnaise
- Non Fat Milk
- Salsa
- Sliced Turkey Breast (for snacks)
- Whole Wheat Bread, Best from Great Harvest Bread Co. If not, Wheat or Oat Bread from the grocery store
- Zucchini (fresh)
- Tomato (fresh)
- Broccoli (fresh)

Protein/Calorie Counter

KEY:

Cal = Calories   Pro = Protein in grams

T = Tablespoon   t = teaspoon

oz = ounce

FOOD	PORTION SIZE	PROTEIN/grams	CALORIES
A			
Alcoholic drinks Gin, Rum, Vodka, Whiskey	3 oz.	0	220
Almonds	1 oz.	6.0	170
Apple, raw	1 medium	0.3	81
Applesauce	½ cup	0	90
Apple juice	½ cup.	0.05	58
Apricots, canned	4 halves	0.5	75
Asparagus, canned	½ cup	2.6	23
Avocado, Florida	1 med. 5"	4.8	340
B			
Bacon, broiled	3 slices	5.8	109
Banana	1 med.	1.2	105
Beans, cooked, red, black	1 cup	15.2	227
Beans, Lima	1 cup	14.6	229
Beans, green, canned	½ cup	0.8	14
Beans, refried	½ cup	6	100
Beef, sirloin steak, broiled, no bone	3.5 oz.	27.6	269
Beef, sirloin steak, broiled, no bone	7.0 oz.	55.2	538
Hamburger, lean	3.5 oz.	24.7	272
Hamburger, lean	7.0 oz.	49.4	544
Beer	12 oz. can	1.1	146
Beets, canned	½ cup	0.8	26
Blueberries, raw	1 cup	1.0	81
Bread, white	1 slice	3.0	100
Bread, wheat	1 slice	4.0	90
Broccoli, fresh	½ cup	2.3	22
Butter, salted	1 T.	0.1	108
C			
Cabbage, cooked	1/2 cup	0.8	17
Cake, choc, choc icing	cupcake	2.2	172
Cake, Pound cake	1 ounce	1.5	131
Carrots, cooked	½ cup	0.9	35
Celery, raw	1 large stalk	0.3	6
Cereal, corn flakes	1 cup	2.0	120
Cereal, oatmeal,	½ cup	5.0	150
Cookies with salt	1 cup	6.1	145
Cheese, American	1 slice	6.3	106

Cheese, Cheddar	1 slice	7.1	114
Chicken, light meat, Roasted, no bone	3.5 oz.	30.9	173
Chicken, dark meat, roasted, no bone	3.5 oz.	27.4	205
Chocolate with nuts	1.5 oz.	4.5	228
Chocolate	1.5 oz.	3.2	233
Coca Cola	12 oz. can	0	145
Cocoa, dry powder	1 T	1.0	11
Coffee, instant	1 tsp.	0.2	4
Coffee, regular brewed	6 oz.	0.2	4
Coffee rich, liquid	1 T.	0	22
Cookies, van. Wafers	7	1.4	125
Cool Whip	2 T.	0	25
Corn, regular canned	½ cup	2	66
Cottage Cheese	4 oz.	14.1	117
Cranberry juice cocktail	6 oz.	0	108
Half and Half Cream	1 T	0.4	20
Cream Cheese	1 T	1.0	45

E

Egg, whole	1 large	6.3	78

F

Fish, fillet cooked	3 oz.	21.1	100
Fruit cocktail, canned	½ cup	0.5	93

G

Ginger ale	12 oz. can	0	124
Grape juice	8 oz.	1.4	154
Grapes, seedless	1 cup	0.6	58
Grapefruit juice, fresh	8 oz.	1.2	96
Grapefruit	Half	0.8	39
Guava, raw	3 oz.	0.7	46

H

Ham, lean, no bone	3.5 oz.	24.9	170

I

Ice Cream	1 cup	8.4	464

L

Lemon Juice, fresh	2 T.	0.2	8
Lettuce, iceberg type	¼ head	0.9	10
Liver, beef, fried	3.5 oz.	26.7	217
Lobster, cooked	3 oz.	17.4	83

M

Macaroni, cooked plain	1 cup	6.7	197
Macaroni and cheese	9.5 oz	12.0	320
Mango, 1 medium	10 oz.	1.1	135
Margarine, salted	1 T.	0	100
Marshmallows	4 regular	0.4	92
Mayonnaise	1 T.	0.2	100
Melon, cantaloupe	1 cup	1.4	56
Milk, whole	8 oz.	8.0	150
Milk, nonfat	8 oz.	8.4	86

Milk, evaporated	8 oz.	16.0	320
Milk, soy	8 oz.	6.6	79
Milk, coconut	1 cup	4.6	445
Milk, condensed	8 oz.	24.0	1040
Molasses	2 T.	0	53
Mushrooms, raw chopped	½ cup	0.7	9
Mustard, prepared	1 t.	1.0	5

O

Oil, any kind	1 cup	0	2000
Olives, black	10	0	90
Olives, green	10	0	40
Onions, chopped	½ cup	0.9	30
Orange	1 medium	1.3	60
Orange juice, fresh	8 oz.	1.7	112
Oysters, raw	6 medium	4.4	50

P

Papaya, raw	1 medium	1.9	119
Papaya nectar	8 oz.	0.4	143
Peach nectar	8 oz.	0.7	134
Peaches, canned	1 cup	1.2	189
Peach, raw, med	3 oz.	0.6	37
Peas, frozen	2/3 cup	5	70
Peanut Butter	2 T.	7.7	188
Peanuts, salted	1 oz.	7.0	160
Pear nectar	8 oz.	0.3	150
Pears, canned	1 cup	0.5	189
Pear, fresh, medium	5 oz.	0.6	98
Peas, green, canned	½ cup	3.5	62
Pecans, roasted	1 oz.	2.3	187
Pepsi cola	12 oz. can	0	50
Pickles, dill	1 large	0.4	12
Pie, apple, frozen	1/8 pie	2.4	296
Pie, cherry, frozen.	1/8 pie	2.5	325
Pie, pumpkin, frozen.	1/8 pie	4.3	229
Pineapple, canned	1 cup	0.9	199
Pineapple juice	8 oz.	0.8	140
Pineapple raw, chopped	1 cup	0.6	76
Pizza, cheese	1/8 of 12"	7.7	140
Pizza, cheese/meat	1/8 of 12"	13.0	184
Pork roast loin, no bone	3.5 oz	27.6	199
Potato, baked	med. 7 oz.	4.6	220
Potato, fries, frozen.	10 strips	1.7	109
Potato, instant	1 cup	4.0	238
Prune juice	8 oz.	1.6	182
Prunes, dried	10	2.2	201
Pudding, instant choc	½ cup	4.4	158

R

Raisins	2/3 cup	3.4	302
Rice, white, cooked	1 cup	4.0	170
Rice, wild, cooked	1 cup	6.5	166

S

Salad dressing:			
Blue Cheese (Light)	2 T.	2.0	140
French	2 T.	0	42
Italian	2 T.	0	32
Ranch	2 T.	1.0	60
Thousand Island	2 T.	0.2	48
Sausage, bologna slice	1 oz.	2.8	72
Sausage, frankfurter	1 - 2 oz	6.8	180
Sausage, pork link	2 oz.	10.8	256
Sherbet, orange	1 cup	2.2	264
Shrimp, cooked	3 oz.	17.8	84
Shrimp, breaded/fried	3 oz.	18.2	206
Soup, chicken veg.	1 cup	12.3	166
Soup, chicken noodle	1 cup	12.0	160
Soup, veg. Campbell's	1 cup	3.5	122
Soup, veg. beef	1 cup	10.9	96
Soup, cream mushroom	1 cup	4.3	77
Sour cream	2 T.	0.8	52
Sour cream, fat free	2 T.	0	35
Soy Sauce	1 T.	1.5	11
Soybeans, boiled	1 cup	28.6	298
Squash, baked mashed	1 cup	2.2	114
Squash, zucchini	1 cup	1.2	28
Strawberries, fresh	1 cup	0.9	45
Sugar, white	1 T.	0	50
Sweet potato, baked	4 oz.	2.0	117

T

Tamarind, 1 med.	3 oz.	0.5	37
Tea, prepared brewed	1 cup	0	2
Tofu, raw	1 cup	20.0	188
Tomato, medium	4 oz.	1.0	26
Tomato, canned	1 cup	2.0	80
Tomato, paste	2 T	2.0	30
Tomato juice	6 oz.	1.4	31
Tuna, solid in oil	3 oz.	22.6	158
Tuna, solid in water	3 oz.	21.7	99
Turkey, breast roasted.	3.5 oz.	22.2	126

V

Vegetables, mixed frozen (carrots, corn, peas, green beans, lima beans)	½ cup	2.6	59
Vinegar, cider	1 T.	0	2

W

Waffle, frozen 4" sq.	1	2.0	87
Walnuts, English	14 halves	4.1	182
Watermelon	1 cup	1.0	51
Wine, white	3.5 oz.	0.1	70
Wine, red	3.5 oz.	0.2	74

Y

Yogurt, plain Dannon	8 oz.	11.0	140
Yogurt, fruit Yoplait	6 oz	7.0	180

Yogurt, frozen, Sundae Hot Fudge McDonalds	1	7.3	240
Wine, white	3.5 oz.	0.1	70
Wine, red	3.5 oz.	0.2	74

FAST FOODS

These Foods are high in Fat, Potassium, Sodium and Phosphorus.. By listing them, we are not endorsing them. We are only demonstrating their high caloric, fat, and salt content. With good judgment, you can occasionally, selectively, choose some safe items, such as Wendy's broiled chicken sandwich, made especially for you with mustard, lettuce, pickle and tomato only.

Burger King

Food Item	Protein	Calories
Whopper	27.0	640
Cheeseburger	23.0	380
Croissandwich, Sausage, ham and cheese	22.0	600
Chicken Sandwich	26.0	710
Medium French Fries	5.0	370
Onion Rings	4.0	310
Apple Pie	3.0	300
Chocolate Shake, medium	9.0	320

Kentucky Fried Chicken

Baked Chicken BBQ Baked Beans 5.5 oz.	6.0	190
Biscuit 2 oz.	4.0	180
Chicken, original recipe Breast 5.4 oz.	29.0	400
Chicken, original recipe Leg 2.2 oz.	13.0	140
Chicken, original recipe Thigh 3.2 oz.	16.0	250
Chicken, original recipe Wing 1.6 oz.	9.0	140
Macaroni and cheese 5.4 oz.	7.0	180
Chicken, Extra Crispy Breast 5.9 oz.	31.0	470
Chicken, Extra Crispy Leg 2.4 oz.	13.0	190
Chicken, Extra Crispy Thigh 4.2 oz.	19.0	370
Chicken, Extra Crispy Wing 1.9 oz.	10.0	210
Potatoes, mashed/gravy 4.8 oz.	1.0	120
Corn Bread 2 oz.	3.0	228

McDonalds

Cheeseburger	15.0	310
Quarter Pounder	23.1	410
Quarter Pounder with Cheese	28.5	520
Chicken McNuggets, 1 serving	19.0	290

Big Mac	25.2	560
Fish Fillet Sandwich	13.8	440
French Fries, Regular	11.3	570
Egg McMuffin	18.2	290
Hotcakes and Syrup	8.2	410
Scrambled Eggs	12.4	140
Sausage	8.4	180
Apple Pie	2.2	260
Hot Fudge Sundae, frozen. yogurt	7.3	240
Choc. Shake	11.6	320
Chef's Salad, no dressing	20.5	230
Chef's Salad, Ranch dressing, 0.5 oz.	0.2	83
Chunky Chicken Salad	23.1	140
Chunky Chicken Salad,		
Blue cheese dressing, 0.5oz	0.5	70

Pizza Hut

BIG FOOT Cheese 1 slice, 2.7 oz.	10.0	186
BIG FOOT Pepperoni 1 slice, 2.8 oz.	10.0	205
PAN PIZZA Beef 4.2 oz., 1 slice	14.0	286
PAN PIZZA Cheese 3.8 oz., 1 slice	12.0	261
PAN PIZZA Supreme, 5.1 oz.,1 slice	15.0	323
THIN'N CRISPY PIZZA Italian		
Sausage 3.3 oz., 1 slice	11.0	236
THIN'N CRISPY PIZZA Pepperoni,		
3 oz., 1 slice	11.0	215
THIN'N CRISPY PIZZA Cheese		
3.0 oz., 1 slice	11.0	205

Taco Bell

Burrito, 1 bean	13.0	373
Chili Cheese, Burrito	14.3	326
Light Chicken Burrito	18.3	309
Fajita, 1 chicken	17.8	461
Fajita, 1 steak	9.9	465
Supreme Chicken Fajita	18.6	505
Taco, 1	10.2	183
Pico de gallo sauce, 1 serving.	0.2	7
Salsa, 1 serving	0.9	24

Wendy's

Chicken Breaded Sandwich	28.0	440
Stuffed Pita Chicken Caesar 8.4 oz	36.0	490
Stuffed Pita Classic Greek 8.25 oz.	17.0	430
Baked Potato, Cheese and Bacon	17.0	540
Baked Potato, Chili and Cheese	20.0	620
Chicken Nuggets	14.0	210
Bar-B-Q Nugget Sauce	1.0	50
Bar-B-Q Honey Sauce	0	130

Use the *"chart"*. It will help you track all food intake. You will need to make a few copies. We have included ten pages to get you started, and a sample chart already filled in. The sample chart is located after the three blank charts. Do not attempt to start filling out the chart until you have completed reading and understanding the whole program.

The reason to keep the diary is to heighten your awareness of what you put in your mouth, making you more likely to consider low-fat selections with quality carbohydrates and adequate protein. Also, if you know what your daily allotment of calories are, you will know when you have reached it, and when to stop eating. Finally, the average American has a very narrow range of food choices. If you count calories for just two to three weeks, you will know what calories, fat, protein 90% of all the food you eat contain. You will need to make copies of the chart for each day of the week.

Calculate your daily caloric and protein requirements

Resting Metabolic Rate (RMR)	
Caloric expenditure today from exercise	+
Total caloric expenditure today	=
Minus 500 calories for 1 lb per week fat loss	-
TOTAL: Caloric intake goal for today	=
TOTAL: Protein goal for today	

Design your personalized nutritional program

Now, go forward and fill in a daily menu plan on the chart. You can do this in advance to help conserve calories, or you can do it as you go. If you do it as you go, be sure and keep a running total so you will know when you have reached your goal.

You are an athlete now and no longer a couch potato. Therefore, be sure and set your daily program based around the correct number of grams of protein. Then, fill the balance with high quality carbohydrates and the natural fats that foods contain. If you are running too low on fat, add a half an avocado. Sauté your veggies in a tablespoon of olive oil. Now, go for it and get the body you have dreamed about.

Splurging is allowed.
If you start to feel deprived, you will eventually just say, forget the whole

thing as you have done before. If you can stick to the plan all week, you can splurge on the weekends by going off track for <u>one or two meals only</u>. However, try not to ruin in two meals what you worked so hard to accomplish all week. Use your head, but cheating is allowed. Eventually, that splurging will be isolated to an occasional dessert or high glycemic index carbohydrate with lunch or dinner. By then, your metabolism will be revving to a point that those occasional few extra calories won't have an affect.

Remember, if you are going to have your "cheat meal", be sure and drink a full 8 ounce glass of water first, <u>with no ice</u>.

Date:_____   Day of the week:_____

Caloric goal:_____   Protein goal:_____

Food or Beverage	Portion	Calories	Protein
Breakfast – Time am			
Snack – Time am			
Lunch – Time pm			
Snack – Time pm			
Dinner – Time pm			
Daily Totals:			

Date:_____   Day of the week:_____

Caloric goal:_____   Protein goal:_____

Food or Beverage	Portion	Calories	Protein
Breakfast – Time am			
Snack – Time am			
Lunch – Time pm			
Snack – Time pm			
Dinner – Time pm			
Daily Totals:			

The following is a sample daily menu for a female whose total daily caloric goal is 1,291 calories with 95 grams of protein. It is a lot of food.
If you are male and need additional calories and protein, add the bold line items to your chart, and you will end up with 1826.5 Calories and 174.8 grams of protein.

Food or Beverage	Portion	Calories	Protein
BREAKFAST -- AM			
Nutrigrain Cereal	1 1/3 cup	180	6
Non-fat milk	½ cup	43	4.2
Banana	1/2		
OR Kip's cereal concoction	1 ½ cup	190	10
Protein shake made with 8 oz skim milk	**16 oz**	**206**	**30.4**
SNACK -- AM			
Premier Protein bar from Costco	½	140	15.5
Premier Protein bar from Costco	**½**	**140**	**15.5**
LUNCH -- Turkey Sandwich			
Sliced Turkey	4 oz	126	22
Sliced Turkey	**2 oz**	**63**	**11**
Whole wheat bread	2 slices	180	8
Lettuce	1 leaf	0	0
Tomato	2 slices	5	0
Non-fat mayo. or mustard	0	0	0
SNACK -- PM			
Apple	1	81	.3
DINNER -- PM			
Red wine	7 oz	148	.4
Broiled or grilled chicken breast, no skin	3.5 oz	126	22
Broiled or grilled chicken breast, no skin	**3.5 oz**	**126**	**22**
Broccoli, steamed with no butter (a lot)	9 oz	42	4.5
Applesauce	½ cup	90	0
Skim milk	12 oz	129	13
Daily Totals:		**1,291.5**	**95.4**
Alternate Daily Totals:		**1,826.5**	**174.8**

Recipes

Chicken with Cilantro Pesto

Pesto:
2 tablespoons olive oil
2 teaspoons lemon juice
1/4 cup grated fresh Parmesan cheese
2 cloves garlic
1 cup firmly packed fresh cilantro
1/4 cup reduced sodium chicken broth

1 pound boneless, skinless chicken breast (approx. 3 breasts)
1 tablespoon olive oil
1 1/2 cups sliced asparagus (approx. 1/2 pound)
1 cup fresh mushrooms, sliced
1 medium onion, chopped
8 cups cooked pasta (approx. 4 cups uncooked)

Place all pesto ingredients except broth into a blender or food processor. Cover and pulse blend. Add just enough broth if needed to make a paste.

Cut chicken into bite-sized pieces. Heat oil in a large nonstick skillet over medium heat. Add chicken breast, onion and mushrooms. Cook about 8 minutes or until chicken is no longer pink.

Cook pasta according to package directions. Add sliced asparagus during the last 2 minutes of cooking. Drain pasta and add to chicken mixture. Add pesto and toss to coat.

Makes 8 Servings
Serving Size: 12 ounces

Nutrients per serving:
Calories: 339
Total fat: 8 grams (21% of calories)
Saturated fat: 1 gram
Cholesterol: 35 mg
Sodium: 95 mg
Carbohydrate: 44 grams (52% of calories)
Protein: 23 grams (27% of calories)
Dietary fiber: 3 grams

Garden Clam Chowder

1 cup small shells or other small pasta
3 cups reduced fat milk
1 (10 ounce) bag frozen mixed vegetables, thawed and drained
1/2 teaspoon dried thyme
1/2 teaspoon paprika
1 1/2 teaspoon cornstarch
1 (6 ounce) can clams, drained
Salt and pepper to taste

Prepare pasta according to package directions and drain. Rinse pasta under cold water to cool. Combine 2 1/2 cups milk, vegetables, thyme, paprika and pasta in a saucepan. Cook over medium heat until hot but not boiling. Combine remaining 1/2-cup milk and cornstarch and mix until cornstarch dissolves. Stir cornstarch into soup and return to simmer. Add clams and simmer for 3 minutes. Season with salt and cracked black pepper.

Makes 4 Servings
Serving Size: 12 ounces

Nutrients per serving:
Calories: 256
Total fat: 3 grams (11% of calories)
Saturated fat: 1 gram
Cholesterol: 22 mg
Sodium: 152 mg
Carbohydrate: 40 grams (62% of calories)
Protein: 17 grams (27% of calories)
Dietary fiber: 4 grams

Halibut Kabobs

1 pound halibut steaks (or other white fish), 1 inch thick
1 medium zucchini
1 medium yellow squash
1 large purple onion
12 cherry tomatoes
1/2 teaspoon sugar
2 clove garlic, finely chopped
3 tablespoons reduced sodium soy sauce
1 teaspoon ginger root, grated
1 teaspoon sesame oil
1 tablespoon sesame seeds

Cut fish, zucchini and squash into 3/4 inch pieces. Quarter onion into similar size pieces. Alternate fish, zucchini, squash, onion and cherry tomatoes on 4 skewers. If using wooden skewers soak in water for 30 minutes to prevent burning. Set oven to broil or barbecue to medium heat.

Combine remaining ingredients and brush generously on all sides of kabobs. Generously spray broiler pan or barbecue grill with nonstick cooking spray. Place kabobs on broiler pan or grill rack about 4 inches from heat. Broil or grill for 2 minutes per side. Turn and baste with remaining marinade during cooking. Total cooking time should be about 6-8 minutes or until fish flakes easily with a fork. Discard any remaining marinade.

Makes 4 Servings
Serving Size: 1 skewer (approx. 4 ounces fish)

Nutrients per serving:
Calories: 194
Total fat: 5 grams (24% of calories)
Saturated fat: 1 gram
Cholesterol: 36 mg
Sodium: 519 mg
Carbohydrate: 10 grams (21% of calories)
Protein: 26 grams (55% of calories)
Dietary fiber: 3 grams

Wonton Soup

1/2 pound ground pork tenderloin
8 medium shrimp, chopped
1 teaspoon chopped ginger root
1 teaspoon reduced sodium soy sauce
1 tablespoon minced cilantro
24 wonton wrappers
32 ounces low sodium chicken broth
32 ounces no-salt added chicken broth
2 green onions, thinly sliced

Heat a large nonstick skillet over medium-high heat until hot. Add ground pork and brown until no longer pink. Add chopped shrimp, ginger root, soy sauce and cilantro and cook 3-5 minutes or until shrimp is no longer opaque. Cool slightly.

Place a small amount of water in a bowl to use for sealing wontons. Place 1 teaspoon filling in the center of each wonton wrapper. Moisten edges with water, fold top corner of wonton wrapper over filling and press firmly to seal.

Hold filled wonton by the tip of the triangle. Gently wrap corners around filling, moisten with water and gently pinch to seal. Set wontons aside on a plate and continue with remaining wontons.

Place broth in a large pot and bring to a light boil. Add wontons one or two at a time and cook until they float, about 1 or 2 minutes. Add green onion and serve.

Makes 6 Servings
Serving Size: 4 wontons and 8 ounces broth

Nutrients per serving:
Calories: 178
Total fat: 3 grams (15% of calories)
Saturated fat: 1 gram
Cholesterol: 40 mg
Sodium: 662 mg
Carbohydrate: 21 grams (42% of calories)
Protein: 21 grams (43% of calories)
Dietary fiber: 1 gram

Garlic Steak for One

1 small, extra lean steak, 4 oz.
2 tablespoons Worcestershire sauce
1 clove garlic, sliced into 10 pieces
Salt and pepper, if desired

Poke holes all over steak with fork, then make 10 little slivers with knife. Put garlic slices into slivers. On plate or in plastic bag, marinate steak in Worcestershire sauce at least 1 hour, turning once, in refrigerator. Away from direct flame, grill or broil steak until done to your liking, turning at least once. Do not char. Add salt and pepper, if desired.

Makes 1 serving
Serving size: 1 (4 ounce) steak

Nutrients per serving:
Calories: 203
Total fat: 8 grams (27% of calories)
Saturated fat: 3 grams
Cholesterol: 68 mg
Sodium: 387 mg
Carbohydrate: 7 grams (15% of calories)
Protein: 24 grams (58% of calories)
Dietary fiber: 0 grams

Tuna Patties with Lemon-Dill Sauce

1 (12 ounce) can tuna packed in water, drained and finely flaked
2 slices whole wheat bread
1/4 cup minced green onion
1/4 cup egg substitute
1/2 cup skim milk
1/2 teaspoon grated lemon peel
1/8 teaspoon garlic powder

Lemon Dill Sauce:
3/4 cup nonfat chicken broth
1/4 cup lemon juice
1 teaspoon dried dill weed

Toast bread and allow to completely cool. Tear toasted bread and place in a blender of food processor and process into crumbs. In large bowl, combine tuna, breadcrumbs, green onion, egg substitute, milk, lemon peel and garlic powder. Form into 4 patties. Spray a large nonstick skillet with cooking spray and heat over medium heat. Cook patties, until golden brown on both sides, about 3 minutes per side.

Sauce: combine all ingredients in a small saucepan and heat over low heat until warm. Add a small amount of flour or cornstarch with a whisk to thicken if desired.

Makes 4 Servings
Serving Size: 1 patty and 2 ounces sauce

Nutrients per serving:
Calories: 162
Total fat: 1 gram (8% of calories)
Saturated fat: trace
Cholesterol: 26 mg
Sodium: 517 mg
Carbohydrate: 11 grams (27% of calories)
Protein: 26 grams (65% of calories)
Dietary fiber: 1 gram

Caesar Chicken Sandwich

3 tablespoons all-purpose flour
1/2 teaspoon ground pepper
4 (4 ounce) boneless, skinless chicken breasts
6 tablespoons lemon juice
4 cloves garlic, minced
4 teaspoons Worcestershire sauce
Dash hot pepper sauce
2 tablespoons walnuts, chopped
4 teaspoons grated Parmesan cheese
4 reduced fat sandwich rolls
4 leaves romaine lettuce

Combine flour and pepper. Coat chicken with flour mixture and shake off
excess. Spray a nonstick skillet with cooking spray and heat over a
medium heat until hot. Add chicken and lightly brown on both sides.
Combine lemon juice, garlic, Worcestershire and hot pepper sauce and
pour over chicken.

Cover and simmer for 7 minutes on each side or until chicken is no
longer pink. Sprinkle chicken with walnuts and parmesan. Arrange lettuce
on rolls, place chicken on the lettuce and serve.

Nutrients per serving:
Calories: 278
Total fat: 5 grams (16% of calories)
Saturated fat: 1 gram
Cholesterol: 67 mg
Sodium: 349 mg
Carbohydrate: 27 grams (38% of calories)
Protein: 33 grams (46% of calories)
Dietary fiber: 3 grams

Pasta e Fagioli

8 ounces small pasta
2 teaspoon olive oil
1/2 cup chopped onion
2 garlic cloves, minced
1/2 pound ground turkey breast
1-2 teaspoons dried oregano
Freshly ground black pepper, to taste
3 cups fat-free, reduced sodium chicken broth
1 (28 ounce) can crushed tomatoes
2 (15 ounce) cans white kidney beans, rinsed and drained
1/4 cup grated Parmesan cheese

Cook pasta according to package directions. Drain and set aside.
Meanwhile, in large stockpot, heat oil over medium heat. Add onion and
garlic and sauté 3 minutes, until soft. Add turkey and cook 5 minutes,
until meat is browned, breaking up meat as it cooks. Add oregano and
black pepper; stir to coat. Add broth, tomatoes and beans and bring
mixture to boil. Reduce heat, cover and simmer 10 minutes. Stir in
cooked pasta and heat through. Ladle mixture into bowls and top with
Parmesan cheese.

Makes 8 servings
Serving size 1 cup

Nutrients per serving:
Calories: 289
Total fat: 4 grams (12% of calories)
Saturated fat: 1 gram
Cholesterol: 20 mg
Sodium: 587 mg
Carbohydrate: 46 grams (61% of calories)
Protein: 19 grams (27% of calories)
Dietary fiber: 9 grams

Macaroni and Cheese

1 1/2 tablespoons reduced calorie margarine
1/4 cup all-purpose flour
3/4 teaspoon dry mustard
1/8 teaspoon ground red pepper
3 cups nonfat milk
1 1/4 cups shredded reduced fat cheddar cheese
1/4 cup shredded reduced fat Swiss cheese
5 cups cooked elbow macaroni, cooked without salt or fat

Preheat oven to 350 degrees. Melt margarine in a small saucepan over medium heat. Add flour and mix well. Add milk and mix with wire whisk over low heat, stirring continuously. Add dry mustard and ground red pepper and cheeses, mix and continue to heat over low heat until cheese is melted.

Pour pasta into a glass-baking dish, add cheese sauce and toss to coat. Season with salt and pepper and bake uncovered at 350 degrees for about 35 minutes or until heated through.

Makes 8 Servings
Serving Size: 6 ounces

Nutrients per serving:
Calories: 238
Total fat: 5 grams (20% of calories)
Saturated fat: 2 grams
Cholesterol: 12 mg
Sodium: 186 mg
Carbohydrate: 33 grams (56% of calories)
Protein: 14 grams (23% of calories)
Dietary fiber: 1 gram

Chicken and Black Bean Enchiladas

Nonstick cooking spray
1/2 (15 ounce) can black beans, rinsed and drained (approximately 1/2 cup)
2 teaspoons chili powder
1 teaspoon ground cumin
1 pickled jalapeño, minced, optional
1 cup prepared salsa
4 (8-inch) flour tortillas
1 cup cooked shredded chicken breast
2 oz. shredded reduced fat Monterey Jack cheese
1/2 cup chopped scallions

Preheat oven to 400 degrees. Coat shallow baking pan with cooking spray and set aside. In large bowl, combine beans, chili powder, cumin, jalapeño and 1/2 cup of salsa. Mash with fork until blended. Spoon mixture onto center of each tortilla. Place chicken over bean mixture. Roll up tortillas, fold in ends and place side by side in bottom of prepared pan. Top with salsa, cheese and scallions. Cover with foil and bake 20 minutes. Uncover and bake 10 more minutes, until cheese is golden.

Makes 4 servings.
Serving size: 1 enchilada

Nutrients per serving:
Calories: 361
Total fat: 8 grams (21% of calories)
Saturated fat: 3 grams
Cholesterol: 45 mg
Sodium: 741 mg
Carbohydrate: 44 grams (52% of calories)
Protein: 26 grams (26% of calories)
Dietary fiber: 8 grams

Vegetable Minestrone

1/4 cup diced onion
1/4 cup diced celery
1/4 cup diced mushrooms
1/2 cup canned, Italian-style diced tomatoes
1 cup canned white beans, rinsed and drained
2 tablespoons elbow macaroni
2 cups fat-free, reduced sodium chicken or vegetable broth
1/4 teaspoon basil
1/4 teaspoon oregano
Salt and pepper, to taste (optional)

In medium saucepan, combine all ingredients except salt and pepper.
Bring to boil, then reduce heat and simmer, covered, 15 minutes. Season
with salt and pepper, if desired.

Makes 2 servings
Serving Size: 1/2 of recipe

Nutrients per serving:
Calories: 206
Total fat: less than 1 gram (3 % of calories)
Saturated fat: less than 1 gram
Cholesterol: 0 mg
Sodium: 686 mg
Carbohydrate: 39 grams (72% of calories)
Protein: 13 grams (26% of calories)
Dietary fiber: 8 grams

Honey Mustard Salmon with Lime and Pepper

1 tablespoon lime juice
2 teaspoon honey
1 teaspoon prepared mustard
1 salmon fillet, 4-5 ounces
1/4 small yellow pepper, cut in slices
1/4 small red pepper, cut in slices
1/4 small green pepper, cut in slices
Salt and pepper, to taste (optional)

Preheat oven to 400 degrees. In small bowl, mix together first 3 ingredients. Place salmon on piece of parchment paper large enough to fold over and completely cover fish. Poke holes into fish with fork. Pour lime marinade over fish, then top with pepper slices. Add salt and pepper, if desired. Wrap fish in parchment paper, then wrap in tin foil to cover. Bake until done, about 20 minutes.

Makes 1 serving

Nutrients per serving:
Calories: 227
Total fat: 8 grams (19% of calories)
Saturated fat: 1 gram
Cholesterol: 66 mg
Sodium: 117 mg
Carbohydrate: 17 grams (34% of calories)
Protein: 23 grams (47% of calories)
Dietary fiber: 1 gram

Mediterranean Frittata

2 teaspoons olive oil
4 green onions, chopped
1/2 cup chopped fresh basil
2 medium tomatoes, seeded and chopped
1 medium potato, sliced
2 cups reduced fat egg substitute
1/4 cup grated Parmesan cheese
1/4 cup crumpled feta cheese

Heat 1 teaspoon oil in a large non stick skillet until hot. Add onions, basil and tomatoes and sauté for 2 minutes. Remove from heat and keep warm.

Heat remaining teaspoon oil until hot. Add sliced potatoes and cook until tender, about 4 minutes. Reduce heat and arrange potatoes in a layer in the bottom of the skillet. Combine egg substitute and Parmesan cheese and pour over potatoes.

Sprinkle tomatoes, onion and basil on top and heat over medium-low heat until eggs are thickened, about 3-4 minutes. Sprinkle with feta cheese, slice into 4 wedges and serve.

Makes 4 Servings
Serving Size: 1/4 of frittata

Nutrients per serving:
Calories: 161
Total fat: 6 grams (34% of calories)
Saturated fat: 3 grams
Cholesterol: 12 mg
Sodium: 378 mg
Carbohydrate: 12 grams (30% of calories)
Protein: 14 grams (36% of calories)
Dietary fiber: 2 grams

Stuffed Portobello Mushrooms with Cilantro Pesto

Nonstick cooking spray
8 medium-sized Portobello mushrooms (5-6 inches in diameter)
1 cup zucchini, finely chopped
1 cup carrots, shredded
3 green onions, thinly sliced
4 tablespoons unseasoned breadcrumbs
1/2 cup shredded, reduced-fat mozzarella cheese
Salt and pepper to taste

Spinach-Cilantro Pesto:
1 cup loosely packed spinach leaves
1/4 cup finely chopped cilantro
3 cloves garlic
1/4 teaspoon ground cumin
1 tablespoon fat-free parmesan cheese
2 teaspoons olive oil
2 teaspoons lemon juice
1-2 tablespoons water
Salt and pepper to taste

Combine all pesto ingredients except olive oil, lemon juice and water in a blender and pulse blend until coarsely chopped. Gradually add olive oil and lemon juice until mixture is finely chopped. Add enough water to make a paste. Salt and pepper to taste and use at room temperature. Spinach-Cilantro Pesto is also great with pasta and other vegetables.

Rinse mushrooms well. Gently remove mushroom stems without damaging mushroom cap. Chop mushroom stems and set aside. Spray a large nonstick skillet with cooking spray and heat over medium heat until hot. Add chopped mushrooms stems, zucchini, carrots and green onions and sauté until crisp-tender (8-10 minutes). Stir in breadcrumbs and Pesto and mix well.

Divide mixture and gently pack in a mound on the mushroom caps. Line a baking sheet with aluminum foil and spray with nonstick cooking spray. Arrange mushrooms on pan and roast at 425 degrees until mushrooms are tender, about 15 minutes. Uncover, sprinkle mushrooms with cheese and continue cooking for 5 minutes.

Makes 4 Servings
Serving Size: 2 stuffed mushrooms

Nutrients per serving:
Calories: 193
Total fat: 6 grams (25% of calories)
Saturated fat: 1 gram
Cholesterol: 6 mg
Sodium: 191 mg
Carbohydrate: 26 grams (50% of calories)
Protein: 13 grams (25% of calories)
Dietary fiber: 6 grams

Turkey and Vegetable Pasta

4 cups cooked medium-size pasta (rotini, rigatoni, etc.)
1 slice bread
2 cups broccoli florets
2 carrots, sliced
1 tablespoon reduced fat margarine
1 large onion, diced
2 cloves minced garlic
2 celery stalks, diced
1 tablespoon all-purpose flour
1 (14.5 ounce) can reduced sodium, reduced fat chicken broth
1 teaspoon ground sage
2 cups cooked turkey breast, diced

Lightly toast bread and pulse-blend with blender or food processor into breadcrumbs. Prepare pasta according to package directions. Add broccoli and carrots to water during the last 2 minutes. Drain and set aside.

Melt margarine in large nonstick skillet over medium heat. Add onion, garlic and celery and sauté for 3 minutes. Stir in the flour. Add the chicken broth and sage and mix until flour dissolves. Add turkey and continue to simmer for 1 minute or until heated through. Combine the turkey mixture with pasta, vegetable mixture. Sprinkle with breadcrumbs.

Makes 6 Servings
Serving Size: 16 ounces

Nutrients per serving:
Calories: 259
Total fat: 5 grams (17% of calories)
Saturated fat: 1 gram
Cholesterol: 30 mg
Sodium: 460 mg
Carbohydrate: 36 grams (55% of calories)
Protein: 18 grams (27% of calories)
Dietary fiber: 3 grams

Grilled Teriyaki Albacore

4 (4-ounce) albacore tuna steaks, without skin
3/4 cup reduced sodium teriyaki sauce
3 cloves crushed garlic

Combine all ingredients except tuna in a shallow dish and mix well. Place albacore steaks in marinade and marinate in refrigerator for at least 2 hours. Remove albacore from marinade and discard marinade. Grill over medium heat (or broil) for 5 to 6 minutes on each side or until fish flakes easily with a fork.

Makes 4 Servings
Serving Size: 1 tuna steak

Nutrients per serving:
Calories: 197
Total fat: 6 grams (26% of calories)
Saturated fat: 1 gram
Cholesterol: 43 mg
Sodium: 485 mg
Carbohydrate: 6 grams (14% of calories)
Protein: 29 grams (60% of calories)
Dietary fiber: trace

Chicken Nuggets with Pineapple-Orange Sauce

1/4 cup egg substitute
2 tablespoons nonfat milk
3 1/2 cups crushed cornflakes
3 boneless, skinless chicken breasts, cut into nugget-sized pieces

Pineapple-Orange Dipping Sauce
1 (8 ounce) can crushed pineapple in juice
1 tablespoon cornstarch
1/4 cup orange juice
1/4 cup barbecue sauce

Dipping sauce:
Pour undrained pineapple into a blender and process into a thick puree. Combine pineapple puree and remaining sauce ingredients in a small sauce pan and bring to boil. Reduce heat and until sauce thickens. Remove from heat and set aside.

Preheat oven to 400 degrees. Combine egg substitute and milk in a small bowl and mix well. Place cornflakes in a large plastic bag. Dip a couple pieces of chicken in the egg mixture and then shake with cornflakes to coat. Place coated chicken pieces on a baking sheet that has been sprayed with nonstick cooking spray. Repeat until all chicken pieces have been coated. Bake for 15 minutes or until crispy and no longer pink in the center.

Makes 6 Servings
Serving size: 4 ounces chicken and 2 ounces sauce

Nutrients per serving:
Calories: 375
Total fat: 3 grams (8% of calories)
Saturated fat: 1 gram
Cholesterol: 69 mg
Sodium: 731 mg
Carbohydrate: 55 grams (58% of calories)
Protein: 32 grams (34% of calories)
Dietary fiber: 2 grams

Lemon-Rosemary Chicken

2 teaspoons olive oil
4 (4 ounce) boneless, skinless chicken breasts
8 ounces, reduced sodium chicken broth
1 cup freshly squeezed lemon juice (about 4 lemons)
2 tablespoons honey
2 teaspoons finely grated lemon peel
4 tablespoons chopped fresh rosemary
Salt and pepper to taste

Heat oil in a large nonstick skillet over medium-high heat until hot. Add chicken and quickly brown on both sides. Reduce heat and continue cooking until chicken is no longer pink, about 4 minutes per side. Remove chicken from pan and keep warm.

Add remaining ingredients and mix well. Bring to boil, then reduce heat and simmer for 5 minutes to reduce slightly. You can add a little flour or cornstarch to thicken sauce if desired. Return chicken to the saucepan and heat through.

Makes 4 Servings
Serving Size: 1 breast

Nutrients per serving:
Calories: 202
Total fat: 4 grams (16% of calories)
Saturated fat: 1 gram
Cholesterol: 66 mg
Sodium: 340 mg
Carbohydrate: 15 grams (29% of calories)
Protein: 28 grams (54% of calories)
Dietary fiber: 1 gram

Chicken Tortellini and Roasted Vegetable Salad

3 cups whole medium mushrooms
2 cups cubed zucchini
2 cups cubed eggplant
1 medium red onion, cut into wedges and separated
1 1/2 packages cheese-filled tortellini
6 cups bite sized red leaf or romaine lettuce
2 cups cooked and cubed boneless, skinless chicken breasts (about 1 1/2 pounds before cooking)

Sun-Dried Tomato and Basil Vinaigrette:
4 sun-dried tomato halves, not packed in oil
1/2 cup hot water
1/2 cup low sodium, reduced fat chicken broth
2 teaspoons dried basil
2 tablespoons olive oil
2 tablespoons lemon juice
2 tablespoons water
1 clove garlic, minced
1/4 teaspoon salt
1/4 teaspoon pepper

Sun-Dried Tomato and Basil Vinaigrette:
Place sun-dried tomatoes and hot water in a small container. Let stand about 10-15 minutes or until tomatoes are soft. Combine remaining ingredients in a container with a tight fitting lid. Drain water from tomatoes and add to other ingredients. Finely chop tomatoes, add to other ingredients and shake well. Refrigerate until to ready to use.

Heat oven to 425 degrees. Place mushrooms, zucchini, eggplant and onion in a shallow baking dish and spray generously with cooking spray. Bake 20-25 minutes or until vegetables are browned. Cool to room temperature. Cook tortellini according to package directions, drain and cool to room temperature.

Combine roasted vegetables, tortellini, lettuce and chicken in a large bowl. Drizzle with sun-dried tomato and basil vinaigrette; toss to coat and serve.

Makes 6 Servings
Serving Size: 2 cups
Nutrients per serving:
Calories: 244
Total fat: 7 grams (26% of calories)
Saturated fat: 1 gram
Cholesterol: 61 mg
Sodium: 329 mg
Carbohydrate: 21 grams (33% of calories)
Protein: 25 grams (41% of calories)
Dietary fiber: 5 grams

Now that you know how to eat properly, and you either are on an exercise program or are going to start exercising regularly, please use your athletic club membership to the fullest. It only makes sense to attack the problem at both ends, diet and exercise. The more you exercise properly, the more you will maximize your lean mass. That will result in higher metabolism, and you will be stronger and feel better. Prior to your workout you need to provide your body some fuel to get started. Many people think they will burn more fat by stepping on the treadmill with an empty stomach when in fact the reverse is true – you will burn glycogen from your muscles first! This will lead to a decrease in your lean mass over time. I've seen many clients have low lean mass or loose lean mass because of this. The good news is I've seen them reverse this situation by changing how/when they eat. Keep in mind; we are not talking about going to the buffet bar before walking the dog but a light snack, maybe 100-150 calories, before a strenuous workout. This will help you maintain energy levels and get a better workout too. This snack should contain protein as well as carbohydrates and, if your workout lasts for 2 hours or more, you should consider eating something during your workout also.

For your cardio workout we recommend an elliptical trainer (like the Precor Elliptical Cross Trainer). They have zero impact on the joints and burn just as many calories as the more difficult treadmills. Try it for 20 minutes. Current research says "to increase your cardiovascular fitness level, you need to do a cardiovascular exercise for a minimum of 20 minutes". You should do the cross trainer at a comfortable rate for 20 minutes. At the end of 20 minutes, note the number of total calories you burned. Each week, try to increase the total calories burned by 10 total calories over the 20 minute duration. Before you know it, you may be burning from 250 to 300 calories in 20 minutes. That is great and all that you need. On the other hand, there is some research that indicates you can get just as much caloric expenditure for just doing resistance exercise. That research will follow, and you will have to make the choice on your own. We suggest you do both. Twenty minutes on the cross trainer and 30 minutes doing resistance exercise. Now, all bases are covered.

Don't kid yourself. Delete swimming, walking, the recumbent bike, yoga, and Pilates. Those activities should be considered recreational exercise. You can do those things, but they do not generally contribute to retention or the increasing of your lean mass, nor are they responsible for burning the number of calories that "getting in the gym" will burn. You want your muscles to burn the calories to get you fit. Those other activities are like Golf is to an athletic event. It is fun, soothes the soul and tones you somewhat, but is not part of a "serious fitness program". Don't send us quotes or articles from those supposed experts who talk about a morning walk being exercise and a high calorie burner. Nonsense! Generally, the heavy people you see walking just seem to stay heavy. Walking is a good starter exercise. However, it is not part of a SERIOUS exercise program unless walking is all that you are capable of doing.

We recommend you start your program by hiring a qualified personal trainer and have them spend eight hours with you. This should be one hour per session for 8 sessions. Initially, you need to tell them that you want to work your upper body one day and your legs the other day. They may want to split it up a bit, but if you do it this way you can hit all body parts twice a week if you go to the gym four days a week. The personal trainer needs to be certified by a national organization, not a certification granted by the facility where he/she works. You should even ask for the name and phone number of one of their success stories. Before you put your body in the hands of anyone, you need to know that they are qualified. On the other hand, you'll find certified personal trainers who are fat and clueless. You'll also find fitness instructors who are the epitome of fitness and could teach at a university, yet are not certified. We'll give you an outline on certification, but you need to use your own judgment.

The most highly regarded of all the certifications are probably ACSM (The American College of Sports Medicine) and CSCS (Certified Strength and Conditioning Specialist). They both require a college degree to even apply for the certification. Other certifications are good, such as ACE and AFFA, but don't require the educational background.

Lastly, be a firm believer in "practice what you preach". Would you ever go to a medical doctor who smoked cigarettes? Likewise, you should never go to a personal trainer who is fat or out of shape. Also, relationships are everything. If you don't feel comfortable with the trainer you interview, keep looking. This is important as your selection process should result in a relationship that will motivate you to complete the program that you start out on.

The following couple of segments are research from renowned organizations and persons. From this information, you should be able to get a grasp of what you type of exercise you need and how often you need to do it. The 12 Week Workout Program is only an example of the programs out there. The 12 Week Workout Program was adapted from a program written by an expert in body building but modified to be of better use by an intermediate athletic club member. Likewise the specific exercises have been tailored to easily adapt to the average athletic club equipment.

The following are research papers on exercise to broaden your understanding.

Article I.   **Medicine & Science in Sports & Exercise®**

Volume 30, Number 6 June 1998 Position Stand

The Recommended Quantity and Quality of Exercise for Developing and Maintaining Cardio Respiratory and Muscular Fitness, and Flexibility in Healthy Adults

This pronouncement was written for the American College of Sports Medicine by: Michael L. Pollock, Ph.D., FACSM (Chairperson), Glenn A. Gaesser, Ph.D., FACSM (Co-chairperson), Janus D. Butcher, M.D., FACSM, Jean-Pierre Després, Ph.D., Rod K. Dishman, Ph.D., FACSM, Barry A. Franklin, Ph.D., FACSM, and Carol Ewing Garber, Ph.D., FACSM.

(a) SUMMARY

ACSM Position Stand on the Recommended Quantity and Quality of Exercise for Developing and Maintaining Cardio Respiratory and Muscular Fitness, and Flexibility in Adults. *Med. Sci. Sports Exerc.,* Vol. 30, No. 6, pp. 975-991, 1998. The combination of frequency, intensity, and duration of chronic exercise has been found to be effective for producing a training effect. The interaction of these factors provide the overload stimulus. In general, the lower the stimulus the lower the training effect, and the greater the stimulus the greater the effect. As a result of specificity of training and the need for maintaining muscular strength and endurance, and flexibility of the major muscle groups, a well-rounded training program including aerobic and resistance training, and flexibility exercises is recommended. Although age in itself is not a limiting factor to exercise training, a more gradual approach in applying the prescription at older ages seems prudent. It has also been shown that aerobic endurance training of fewer than 2 days per week, at less than 40-50% of $V(dot)O_2R$, and for less than 10 min[-1] is generally not a sufficient stimulus for developing and maintaining fitness in healthy adults. Even so, many health benefits from physical activity can be achieved at lower intensities of exercise if frequency and duration of training are increased appropriately. In this regard, physical activity can be accumulated through the day in shorter bouts of 10-min durations.

In the interpretation of this position stand, it must be recognized that the recommendations should be used in the context of participant's needs, goals, and initial abilities. In this regard, a sliding scale as to the amount of time allotted and intensity of effort should be carefully gauged for the cardio respiratory, muscular strength and endurance, and flexibility components of the program. An appropriate warm-up and cool-down period, which would include flexibility exercises, is also recommended. The important factor is to design a program for the individual to provide the proper amount of physical activity to attain maximal benefit at the lowest risk. Emphasis should be placed on factors that result in permanent lifestyle change and encourage a lifetime of physical activity.

(b) INTRODUCTION

Many people are currently involved in cardio respiratory fitness and resistance training programs and efforts to promote participation in all forms of physical activity are being developed and implemented. Thus, the need for guidelines for exercise prescription is apparent. Based on the existing evidence concerning exercise prescription for healthy adults and the need for guidelines, the American College of Sports Medicine (ACSM) makes the following recommendations for the quantity and quality of training for developing and maintaining cardio respiratory fitness, body composition, muscular strength and endurance, and flexibility in the healthy adult:

(i) Cardio Respiratory Fitness and Body Composition

1. Frequency of training: 3-5 $d \cdot wk^{-1}$.

2. Intensity of training: 55/65%-90% of maximum heart rate (HR_{max}), or 40/50%-85% of maximum oxygen uptake reserve ($V(dot)O_2R$) or HR_{max} reserve (HRR).[1] The lower intensity values, i.e., 40-49% of $V(dot)O_2R$ or HRR and 55-64% of HR_{max}, are most applicable to individuals who are quite unfit.

3. Duration of training: 20-60 min of continuous or intermittent (minimum of 10-min bouts accumulated throughout the day) aerobic activity. Duration is dependent on the intensity of the activity; thus, lower-intensity

activity should be conducted over a longer period of time (30 min or more), and, conversely, individuals training at higher levels of intensity should train at least 20 min or longer. Because of the importance of "total fitness" and that it is more readily attained with exercise sessions of longer duration and because of the potential hazards and adherence problems associated with high-intensity activity, moderate-intensity activity of longer duration is recommended for adults not training for athletic competition.

4. Mode of activity: any activity that uses large muscle groups, which can be maintained continuously, and is rhythmical and aerobic in nature, e.g., walking-hiking, running-jogging, cycling-bicycling, cross-country skiing, aerobic dance/group exercise[2]. Rope skipping, rowing, stair climbing, swimming, skating, and various endurance game activities or some combination thereof.

(ii) Muscular Strength and Endurance, Body Composition, and Flexibility

1. Resistance training: Resistance training should be an integral part of an adult fitness program and of a sufficient intensity to enhance strength, muscular endurance, and maintain fat-free mass (FFM). Resistance training should be progressive in nature, individualized, and provide a stimulus to all the major muscle groups. One set of 8-10 exercises that condition the major muscle groups 2-3 $d \cdot wk^{-1}$ is recommended. Multiple-set regimens may provide greater benefits if time allows. Most persons should complete 8-12 repetitions of each exercise; however, for older and more frail persons (approximately 50-60 yr of age and above), 10-15 repetitions may be more appropriate.

Women and Resistance Training

The Right Program Brings Results for Females Who Train

by Gary R. Hunter, Ph.D., CSCS, FACSM

Women can gain a number of vary positive benefits from participating in a well constructed resistance training program. Many women, however, do not put enough effort into their training. They mistakenly believe that training with low weights for high repetitions will achieve optimal increases in energy expenditure, and body composition. The main advantage in resistance training over other forms of training is the ability to progress the resistance. To achieve optimal gains in muscle size and strength. Women must train at a relatively high resistance (usually somewhere between 65 80 percent of maximum) for 6 to 12 repetitions during two to three workouts each week. At least some of these sets each week must be to exhaustion or near exhaustion. Resistance should be increased when a repetition goal (somewhere between six to 12 repetitions) for an exercise is reached.

Although women can definitely increase muscle size, it should be understood that there is little chance of a woman becoming a behemoth and ending up with a body like Arnold Schwarzenegger. Without drug use or some very specialized training is undertaken for many years, women who resistance train normally just become very fit looking. During maturation, women develop much less muscle mass than men. This means that an untrained woman has fewer muscle cells than an untrained man. This is especially the case for the shoulders and arms. Most if not all muscle growth in an adult occurs through increases in size of existing muscle cells, so the total potential for growth in a woman is less than in a man, especially in the arms and shoulders. Other factors may contribute to a slower increase in muscle size in women following a resistance training program, but they are largely unknown. On the average, a woman can expect about a 10 percent increase in muscle size for a muscle that has been resistance trained for three to six months. Strength will normally increase between 30 50 percent. Quite a bit of variability in how much a woman can expect to increase in strength and muscle size exists, with some women increasing in muscle size very little and others increasing as much as 20 percent. Factors such as genetic predisposition, nutrition, general health of the woman and effort put into the training probably contribute to the variation.

Even though women may not have quite as much potential for strength and muscle size improvement as men, they actually may have more to gain from a functional standpoint. Women are much weaker than men. When matched for body size, the average untrained woman is 35 to 45 percent weaker in the arms and shoulders and 10 to 25 percent weaker in the legs and hips than untrained men. Consequently, untrained women generally experience more difficulty in doing daily tasks such as walking, climbing stairs, and carrying children or groceries. Recent research suggests that difficulty in doing these tasks predispose individuals to decreasing free living physical activity. A reduction in physical activity has two very important negatives:

How We React To Exercise

The amount of energy that we expend decreases as we age. This is partly due to a decrease in muscle mass, but it also seems to be partly due to an independent aging effect. Muscle tissue is about three times more metabolically active than fat tissue. It is not unusual for a woman to gain two to four pounds of muscle following four to six months of moderate resistance training, causing energy expenditure at rest to increase 100 kcal or more/day. Further, modest increases in total energy expenditure may occur because of the energy expended during training and increased participation in a more active lifestyle. This may be important for women, especially older women, in maintaining body weight as they get older. It is important to point out that little increases will be gained in muscle or energy expenditure unless intensity and effort are sufficient.

Although increases in muscle and strength occur quite easily during the first eight to sixteen weeks of training, continued increases are normally more difficult to achieve. The more "trained" an individual, the greater the training stimulus needs to be to create changes in strength and muscle size.

Maintaining a sufficient resistance and effort that will cause a muscle to fatigue in six to twelve repetitions is important to achieve optimal progress. Although progress can be made in the early stages of training on only one set / exercise, both empirical and research data suggest continued improvement for the "trained" individual is not only dependent on maintaining a high relative resistance but on multiple sets.

In other words, continued improvement is dependant on a combination of maintaining sufficient intensity / effort and volume of training.

Gains in strength, muscle size, ease of being physically active, and energy expenditure as well as fat losses occur with resistance training. However, it is important to maintain a relatively high intensity and effort in training to achieve these benefits.

Resistance Exercise vs. Aerobics

By Frank Claps, MEd, CSCS

2001 American College of Sports Medicine conference

The more iron you throw around during high-intensity weight training, the more fat you'll burn afterward. According to three studies presented at the 2001 American College of Sports Medicine annual conference, weightlifting elicits a significant excess post exercise oxygen consumption (EPOC) - which can be a marker for burning calories and, hence, fat loss.

One study presented by researchers at the University of Wisconsin (La Crosse) involved seven male recreational weightlifters who performed an intense 31-minute bout of heavy resistance exercise: four circuits of bench presses, power cleans and squats. Each set was performed at the lifter's predetermined 10-rep max and continued until failure. Two-minute rests were allowed between sets, and oxygen measurements were taken 12 times between 34 hours pre-exercise and 49 hours post-exercise.

The data showed significant elevations in EPOC immediately, 14 hours, 19 hours and 38 hours post-exercise. "These results suggest that EPOC following heavy resistance exercise may exceed that following moderate aerobic exercise," the researchers wrote. "Furthermore, the cumulative energy expenditure as a result of EPOC following heavy resistance exercise may exceed the combined total energy expended during and after aerobic exercise."

High intensity may indeed be the way to go for an improved post-exercise burn, agrees another paper presented by researchers from the University of Kansas (Lawrence). In this study, 11 females performed two separate constant sessions involving two sets of 15 repetitions of nine exercises. In one session, the women worked at 45% of their 8RM; in the second, 80%. While energy expenditure was similar in both, a greater EPOC was recorded following the higher-intensity sessions. "If total energy expenditure is an important consideration during exercise, then high-intensity activities should be considered in the exercise prescription," researchers wrote.

Commonly asked exercise questions:

- How many days per week should I workout?
- How many exercises should I do for each body part?
- How many sets and reps should I do?
- Should I lift heavy weights / low reps or light weights / high reps?
- How often should I train each body part?
- Etc. Etc. Etc...

There is really no right or wrong way to workout. You could ask 10 different bodybuilders to explain their workout routine and most likely you would get 10 different answers.

"Everything works, but nothing works forever." That is probably the most important thing to remember for making consistent progress with your workouts. You can follow most any type of workout routine and you will make good progress for the first few weeks (provided that you are getting adequate nutrition, rest, etc.). But generally after a few weeks of following a set workout program your progress will slow down and eventually you will no longer make progress with that routine.

Our bodies are very smart and naturally accommodate stress. Your body will add as little muscle as necessary to get the job done. This is why construction workers get only big enough to handle the exact amount of work they do during a days work and no bigger, even though they are doing physical work all day long.

Adding muscle is a very unnatural thing to your body. You must constantly throw "curve balls" at your muscles to get them to grow. Generally, you will make the best progress for the first 3 weeks of starting a new workout routine. After 3 weeks your body starts to adapt and your progress will slow down.

In the following workout routine there are 4 different, 3-week workout cycles back to back in order to make a 12 week workout program.

This program requires you to workout 4 days per week. Ideally you would workout on Monday, Tuesday, Thursday, and Friday. And rest on Wednesday's and weekends. However, if this doesn't fit your schedule you can workout on other days of the week. Just make sure that you do not workout for more then 2 days in a row before taking a day off.

By doing this you will give your body plenty of time for recuperation and muscle growth. **Muscles do not grow while you are working out; they**

grow while you are resting. Working out will stress and damage your muscles slightly. Then your body reacts by building up the muscles in anticipation of the stress being repeated. Remember, your body will adapt to the load you put on it. Keep varying that load and increasing that load, and your lean mass will increase.

The Workout Routine

Weeks 1, 2, and 3

Monday

20 minutes of cardio

- Squats:
  * do a couple warm up sets first
  * 3 sets of 6 reps (train heavy, but don't train to failure)
  Note: If you have back problems, you may want to substitute squats with the inclined, plate loaded leg press machine.

- Calf raise:
  * 3 sets of 8 reps

- Thigh Extension:
  * 3 sets of 8 reps

- Incline sit ups:
  * 2 sets of 10-20 reps

Tuesday

20 minutes of cardio

- Incline barbell bench press:
  * do a couple warm up sets first
  *3 sets of 5 reps (train heavy, but don't train to failure)

- Seated dumbbell shoulder press:
  * 3 sets of 6 reps

- Bicep cable curls: (from low pulley)
  * 3 sets of 8 reps

- Tricep push downs: (using straight bar attachment)
  * 3 sets of 8 reps

- Bent over dumbbell lateral raises:
  * 3 sets of 8 reps

Thursday

20 minutes of cardio

- Leg press:
  * do a couple warm up sets first
  * 3 sets of 8 reps

- Leg curls:
  * 3 sets of 8 reps

- Wide grip pull downs:
  * 3 sets of 8 reps

- Hyper extensions:
  * 2 sets of 8 reps

- Ab crunch machine:
  * 1 sets of 50 reps

Friday

20 minutes of cardio

- Incline dumbbell bench press:
  * do a couple warm up sets first
  * 3 sets of 8 reps

- Dumbbell side lateral raises:
  * 3 sets of 8 reps

- Bicep dumbbell curls:
  * 3 sets of 8 reps

- Tricep push downs: (with rope attachment)
  * 3 sets of 8 reps

Keep records of the exercises, weights, sets, and reps that you do. Each workout try to beat what you did for your previous workout. With the squat, dead lift, and incline barbell bench press try to add 5 lbs. to the bar each week and do the same number of sets and reps.

Weeks 4, 5, and 6

Monday

20 minutes of cardio

- Seated Cable Rows:
  * do a couple warm up sets first
  * 3 sets of 8 reps

- Seated shoulder shrugs:
  * 3 sets of 10 reps

- Leg extensions:
  * 3 sets of 10 reps

- Leg curls:
  * 3 sets of 10 reps

- Seated calf raise:

- 3 sets of 10 reps

- Incline sit ups:
  * 2 sets of 10-20 reps

Tuesday

(20 minutes of cardio)

- Decline bench press, barbell or machine:
  * do a couple warm up sets first
  * 3 sets of 6 reps (train heavy, but don't train to failure)

- Seated dumbbell shoulder press: (i.e. military press)
  * 3 sets of 8 reps

- Barbell curls:
  * 3 sets of 8 reps

- Lying tricep extensions: (with the EZ bar)
  * 3 sets of 8 reps

- Cable upright rows: (from the low pulley)
  * 3 sets of 10 reps

Thursday

(20 minutes of cardio)

- Leg Press:
  * do a couple warm up sets first
  * 3 sets of 10 reps

- Seated cable rows:
  * 3 sets of 8 reps

- Leg raises:
  * 3 sets of 10 reps

- Crunches::
  * 2 sets of 25+ reps

Friday

20 minutes of cardio

- Flat dumbbell bench press:
  * do a couple warm up sets first
  * 3 sets of 8 reps

- Dumbbell front lateral raises:
  * 3 sets of 8 reps

- Bicep barbell curls:
  * 4 sets of 12 reps

- Tricep push downs: (with V bar attachment)
  * 3 sets of 10 reps

- Close grip pull downs:
  * 3 sets of 10 reps

Keep records of the exercises, weights, sets, and reps that you do. Each workout try to beat what you did for your previous workout. With the decline bench press and the bent barbell row try to add 5 lbs. to the bar each week and do the same number of sets and reps.

Weeks 7, 8, and 9

Monday

20 minutes of cardio

- Squats:
  * do a couple warm up sets first
  * 4 sets of 5 reps (train heavy, but don't train to failure)

- Chin ups:
  * 4 sets of as many reps as you can do

- Pull down ab crunches:

- 3 sets of 10 reps

- Leg raises:
  * 3 sets of 10 reps

Tuesday

20 minutes of cardio

- Flat barbell bench press:
  * do a couple warm up sets first
  * 3 sets of 6 reps (train heavy, but don't train to failure)

- Bent over dumbbell lateral raises:
  * 3 sets of 8 reps

- Dumbbell side lateral raises:
  * 3 sets of 8 reps

- Dumbbell front lateral raises:
  * 3 sets of 8 reps

- Bicep cable curls: (dumbbells)
  * 3 sets of 8 reps

- Tricep push downs: (using straight bar attachment)
  * 3 sets of 10 reps

Thursday

20 minutes of cardio

- Thigh Extension::
  * do a couple warm up sets first
  * 3 sets of 8 reps

- Leg press:
  * 3 sets of 10 reps

- Chest supported row: (i.e. T-bar row, hammer strength seated row, etc.)
  * 3 sets of 10 reps

- Hyper extensions:

- 3 sets of 10 reps

- Pull down ab crunches:
  * 3 sets of 10 reps

Friday

20 minutes of cardio

- Dumbbell bench press on the stability ball:
  * do a couple warm up sets first
  * 3 sets of 10 reps

- Dumbbell shoulder press sitting on the stability ball:
  * 3 sets of 10 reps

- EZ bar bicep curls:
  * 3 sets of 12 reps

- One arm over head dumbbell extensions:
  * 3 sets of 12 reps

- One arm dumbbell rows:
  * 3 sets of 15 reps

Keep records of the exercises, weights, sets, and reps that you do. Each workout try to beat what you did for your previous workout. With the squat, partial dead lift, and flat barbell bench press try to add 5 lbs. to the bar each week and do the same number of sets and reps.

Weeks 10, 11, and 12

Monday

20 minutes of cardio

- Leg press:
  * do a couple warm up sets first
  * 3 sets of 5 reps (train heavy, but don't train to failure)

- Wide grip pull downs:
  * 3 sets of 10 reps

- Incline sit ups:
  * 4 sets of 10 reps

- Leg raises:
  * 4 sets of 12 reps

Tuesday

20 minutes of cardio)

- Dips: (add extra weight if needed)
  * do a couple warm up sets first
  * 5 sets of 5 reps (train heavy, but don't train to failure)

- Chin ups:
  * 4 sets of as many reps as you can do

- Side lateral raises:
  * 4 sets of 8 reps

- Seated dumbbell shoulder press: (i.e. military press)
  * 4 sets of 8 reps

- Bicep dumbbell preacher curls:
  * 5 sets of 8 reps

- Tricep push downs: (using rope attachment)
  * 5 sets of 10 reps

Thursday

20 minutes of cardio

- Squats:
  * 3 sets of 12 reps

- Leg curls:
  * 3 sets of 8 reps

- Leg extensions:
  *3 sets of 8 reps

- Seated cable rows:
  * 3 sets of 8 reps

- Standing calf raise:
  * 3 sets of 10 reps

- Pull down ab crunches:
  * 3 sets of 12 reps

  Friday: (20 minutes of cardio)

- Push ups with feet elevated on the stability ball:
  * 4 sets of as many reps as you can do

- Seated dumbbell shoulder press:
  * 3 sets of 8 reps

- Standing one arm dumbbell curls:
  * 3 sets of 10 reps

(Super set the curls with the over head tricep extensions, you can use the same dumbbell for both exercises. For example, set of curls with one arm, set of curls with the other arm, set of extensions with one arm, set of extensions with the other arm, with no rest in between.)

- One arm over head dumbbell extensions:
  * 3 sets of 8 reps

- Close grip pull downs:
  * 3 sets of 8 reps

Keep records of the exercises, weights, sets, and reps that you do. Each workout try to beat what you did for your previous workout. With the weighted dips and leg press try to add 5 lbs. to the bar each week and do the same number of sets and reps.

Each 3 week cycle is different. You will focus on different exercises during each cycle. This will allow you to make consistent progress over the long term.

Exercise Journal

It is often easier to track your workout if you have a journal. Especially when you are changing your routine and weights as frequently as we recommend.

Fell free to cut out one of the following pages and make a 12 week journal for yourself. Leave the 2nd copy in your book to keep as a reference.

Day Date

Cardio Workout (In the gym)

	Equipment	Duration	Calories
✓	Elliptical Cross Trainer		
✓	Treadmill		

Strength Training

Today's Focus:	Upper Body _____			Lower Body _____		
Muscle Group	**Action or Equipment**	**Set 1** Reps Wt.		**Set 2** Reps Wt.	**Set 3** Reps Wt.	**Set 4** Reps Wt.

Comments:

Day Date

Cardio Workout (In the gym)

	Equipment	Duration	Calories
✓	Elliptical Cross Trainer		
✓	Treadmill		

Strength Training

Today's Focus:	Upper Body _____		Lower Body _____					
Muscle Group	Action or Equipment	Set 1 Reps	Wt.	Set 2 Reps	Wt.	Set 3 Reps	Wt.	Set 4 Reps Wt.

Comments:

Risk to Benefit Ratios

By Tom Venuto

Ken Kinakin recently wrote a book called "Optimal Muscle Training," which is all about biomechanics, anatomy, muscle testing, resistance training technique, and injury prevention. I consider it groundbreaking, because Kikakin did something rarely seen in the mainstream fitness literature: Rather than making sweeping generalizations about exercise safety or usefulness, he analyzed 125 popular weight training techniques and rated them according to risk and benefit.

Understanding risks and benefits enhances your training experience by giving you clearer distinctions, providing you with more choices and helping you make better decisions. For example, some exercises have low risk and high benefit, making them excellent choices for almost anyone. Others have high risk and low benefit, which usually indicates a poor technique best avoided. There are also exercises with high risk and high benefit, which means the exercise, while risky, could have high value to advanced trainees under certain circumstances.

Here's an example: If you asked a typical personal trainer at a health club whether it was okay to perform squats with your heels elevated on a board or wedge, 99% of them would cringe and scream, "That's terrible for you! You'll blow out your knees! NEVER do squats with your heels elevated – always do them flat footed." This is a typical "good or bad" judgment, which neglects to acknowledge the risk to benefit ratio.

The risk is greater stress on the knees. The benefits include greater quad development, less hip involvement, more emphasis placed on the medialis portion of the quadriceps, a more comfortable position for those who lack flexibility, and a more upright torso with less stress on the lower back.

So what does all this have to do with losing fat? Well, I see the same phenomenon among fitness professionals and practitioners alike when it comes to judging the usefulness of fat loss techniques (training or dietary), especially today with the anti-aerobics pendulum having swung all the way to the right.

Many people take an all or none attitude, such as "You should NEVER do cardio on an empty stomach because that causes you to lose muscle" or, "cardio is completely worthless," or "Low carb diets don't work because they deplete your glycogen and kill your energy so you can't train hard. Always eat plenty of carbs."

A better approach would be to analyze each nutrition or training technique according to its risk to benefit ratio (rather than focusing only on risks, and denying that any benefits exist). Just like all strength training activities carry a risk, so do most fat loss techniques. What makes an exercise or nutrition technique worth including in your program is whether the benefits outweigh the risk given your goals and situation.

What I'd like to do is review a group of aggressive, extreme and/or controversial techniques for fat loss which some bodybuilders and fitness enthusiasts embrace as safe and highly effective, while others claim they're worthless, dangerous or counterproductive. By weighing the risks and benefits of each technique, you'll be able to make a much more educated decision about whether to use these techniques yourself.

THE RATING SYSTEM

In Kinakin's book, he outlined a simple three-point rating system with low (1), medium (2) and high (3) risk-benefit ratings, which I have adopted here for fat loss techniques. An exercise that is low risk (1), low benefit (1) might safely provide benefits to a beginner, but would do little for advanced trainees. An exercise with high risk (3) and low benefit (1) shows poor technique with high potential for negative effects (such as muscle loss, overtraining or injury), which are not balanced by any substantial benefits. Low risk (1) and high benefit (3) generally indicates an all-around excellent method with great benefits and virtually no downside. Techniques can also fall somewhere in the middle (medium risk and medium benefit).

After seeing how risks and benefits can be weighed against each other, the lesson becomes clear: Many high risk methods do have applications under the right circumstances - provided the benefit is also high. Kinakin used the skiing analogy to illustrate this point: Ski trails are marked with different colors and labels; the green circle for the beginner trail offers the lowest difficulty and lowest risk of injury, but offers the least benefit or gratification during the experience. The black diamond slopes are for expert skiers with the highest degree of difficulty and highest risk of injury, but they also provide the greatest benefit and gratification during the experience. A beginner to exercise and dieting who hasn't even mastered fundamentals would not be any wiser to use the high risk, "advanced" fat loss or training technique any more than a novice skier would to take a plunge down a black diamond ski slope.

With risk management and careful tracking of results, high-risk fat loss techniques can often be used very successfully. The ratings of each technique that follow will help you decide which ones best apply to you.

THE TECHNIQUES

Fasted cardio in the morning
One of the most controversial fat loss techniques is performing cardio first thing in the morning on an empty stomach. This method is widely embraced by bodybuilders and recommended by many trainers and nutritionists. Other experts claim that the risk of muscle loss is too high and they argue whether workout timing makes any difference in the overall scheme of 24 hour energy expenditure. With low blood sugar and low glycogen levels on awakening, it appears that the body is in a perfect state to burn fat preferentially, but combined with high a.m. cortisol levels, it may also be a perfect state to burn muscle. Therefore, the benefit is high, but so is the risk. Body composition must be carefully monitored when using this technique.
RISK: 3 (high)
BENEFIT: 3 (high)

Cardio in the morning after protein consumption
One of the biggest concerns brought up by opponents of fasted morning cardio is the potential for losing lean body mass. One way to help combat the possible loss of lean body mass is to eat a small protein-only meal or to consume a protein drink (no carbs) immediately upon awakening, then perform the cardio shortly thereafter. This decreases the risk by suppressing cortisol and preventing muscle breakdown, while maintaining the high benefit by keeping your blood sugar and insulin levels low.
RISK: 2 (moderate)
BENEFIT: 3 (high)

Cardio at night
Many bodybuilders and weight loss seekers perform cardio late at night and then do not eat afterward in an attempt to increase fat loss. There are benefits to this method, but they are moderate at best, and the risks are high. Late night training may also keep you awake, disrupting your sleep cycle and recovery. Once you do fall asleep, your metabolic rate decreases rapidly, so you don't reap the full value of the post workout metabolic increase that is achieved with exercise earlier in the day. Risk of muscle loss is high, so body composition must be monitored very closely.
RISK: 3 (high)
BENEFIT: 2 (moderate)

Short duration, high intensity interval training
One of the most popular trends in fitness today is high intensity interval training (HIIT). These workouts consist of short periods of high intensity work intervals followed by short periods of lower intensity recovery intervals. Generally, the intervals are 30 to 120 seconds in length and the total duration is in the 15-25 minute range. Research has shown that HIIT causes a larger increase in post-exercise energy expenditure than moderate intensity, steady-state exercise, which

keeps you burning calories at an elevated rate for an extended period even after the workout is over. There are risks, especially to the beginner, the non-conditioned or the person unaware of his or her health status. However, because intensity is relative to each individual, risk is moderate and easily managed, while the benefits are high. For someone who is already highly fit, the risks are lower.

RISK 2 (moderate)
BENEFIT 3 (high)

Moderate duration, moderate to moderately-high intensity cardio

When cardio is performed for a moderate duration (approx 30 to 45 minutes per session) with the intensity held at the upper end of the "target heart zone," (moderate to moderately-high), large amounts of body fat can be burned during the session. There is also a substantial post exercise elevation in metabolic rate, which, although not as high as that experienced from HIIT, also has a measurable impact on fat loss after the workout.

RISK: 2 (moderate)
BENEFIT: 3 (high)

Long duration, low intensity cardio

Long duration cardio (60 minutes per day or more) does carry the benefit of more calories burned from fat and a moderately high cumulative calorie burn. However, intensity and duration are inversely related, therefore long duration cardio, by nature, is low in intensity. Low intensity cardio, while having the benefit of burning more fat relative to carbs, does not burn as many total calories per unit of time, nor does it have much impact on post exercise energy expenditure. This makes long duration, low intensity cardio (such as walking) most appropriate as a fat loss technique for beginners who can't achieve higher intensities yet. Furthermore, this method is not time efficient. A long walk can be a very good (if not ideal) fat loss method for someone who is unfit, older, overweight, or has orthopedic problems. It also provides great health and even mental benefits. But there is little point in doing an hour or more per session when you can achieve equal if not greater calorie burn and post exercise metabolic increase by doing briefer sessions with higher intensity.

RISK: 1 (low)
BENEFIT: 2 (moderate)

High frequency cardio (5-7 days per week)

Daily cardio performed at a sufficient intensity is considered by many to be a no-brainer fat loss technique for two reasons: First, total caloric expenditure is increased over the course of the week. Since fat loss is a function of calories burned versus calories consumed, increasing cardio activity from three days per week to six days per week, will in theory, double the rate of fat loss in that period. Second, frequent cardio helps maintain metabolic momentum and keeps the metabolism "spinning" by avoiding long periods of inactivity, resulting in metabolic slowdown. These two factors make the benefit of this technique high.

There is moderate risk, however, of overtraining or muscle loss. Risk of aerobic adaptation also increases if the high frequency is maintained over a prolonged period of time. Risks increase relative to the duration of each session and the number of weeks the high volume is maintained. Brief daily sessions have an even more favorable risk to benefit ratio.
RISK: 2 (moderate)
BENEFIT: 3 (high)

High-density weight training (increased volume per unit of time)
Ironically, one of the fat loss techniques with the best risk to benefit ratio has nothing to do with dieting or aerobics. Most bodybuilders decrease their rest intervals between sets and exercises prior to competitions in order to boost intensity, increase hypertrophy, release more growth hormone and simultaneously burn more fat. This is known as high-density training and the goal is to condense more work into less time. The risks are low because even beginners can use the technique, they simply need to adjust the amount of resistance to their strength level. Strength gains are compromised on this type of program, but assuming the goal is fat loss, not strength, that would not be considered a risk. Benefits are highest when the majority of exercises selected are multi-joint movements involving large muscle groups, and/or activating the core and as much of the body as possible. (Note: other forms of high density weight training include supersets, tri sets and giant sets).
RISK: 1 (low)
BENEFIT: 3 (high)

High protein, very low carb, very low fat diets
A very high protein diet that is nearly devoid of carbs AND fat can cause very rapid weight loss, but the risk of muscle loss is extremely high. An example of this diet is the meat/fish and water diet or the slightly less severe lean protein and green veggies diet. This can cause weight and body fat to come off at an alarming rate, but the risks are very high. Risks include loss of lean mass, loss of strength, low energy levels, nutritional deficiencies, impaired mental acuity, dehydration, and rapid weight regain with the reintroduction of carbohydrates.
RISK 3 (high)
BENEFIT 1 (low)

Ketogenic dieting (very low carbs, moderate or high fat)
By eating lean protein with high fat and keeping carbohydrates so low that you enter ketosis (usually 30-70 grams of carbs a day or less), many dieters report reaching levels of leanness they were not able to achieve with any other method. Reducing carbs drastically does seem to accelerate fat loss in virtually any body type, but seems to have greater benefits for those who were hypoglycemic and carb sensitive to begin with. Other people report only moderate fat loss but great losses of energy, weakness, flat muscles and loss of mental acuity. The benefits of low carb diets in general seem to vary from person to person and a major risk, in addition to those already mentioned, is the regain of lost weight with rapid

reintroduction of carbohydrates. A slow transitional period into maintenance decreases the risks. Benefits may be higher if some form of "re-feeding" is employed (such as cyclical ketogenic dieting).
RISK: 2 (moderate)
BENEFIT: 2 (moderate)

Extreme calorie reductions
Many people still believe that severely cutting calories is the best and fastest way to lose body fat. While sharp reductions in calories may cause large and rapid losses of weight, much of the weight loss is often muscle and water, and the risk of long term damage to the metabolism, plateaus and weight re-gain is very high. Some people are consciously aware of the risks, yet they choose to employ severe calorie cutting anyway because they're under time pressure to achieve a fat loss goal. However, the risks are so high and the benefits are so low, it would be more advisable to use a combination of other techniques that offer greater benefits relative to the risks.
RISK: 3 (high)
BENEFIT: 1 (Low)

Avoiding food for 2 to 3 hours before bedtime
Another controversial technique for accelerating fat loss is the avoidance of food for at least two to three hours before bedtime. Increased fat loss is achieved by increasing the length of the nighttime fast (which is broken by "break-fast"). Fat loss is also believed to be increased by avoiding food at a time when activity levels will be low (and the body will not be burning many calories), when glycogen may be topped off from a full day of eating, and when insulin sensitivity is lower. The potential benefit is high, but so is the risk. Body composition must be carefully monitored when using this technique.
RISK: 3 (high)
BENEFIT: 3 (high)

Tapering calories and or carbohydrates
Calorie or carbohydrate tapering involves decreasing carbohydrate portions and or total meal size as the day goes on. This technique works for the same reasons and carries the same risk-benefit ratio as the previous technique. Risk of muscle loss can be reduced by eating a protein-only or protein and fat meal close to bedtime. It's also worth noting that carbs eaten before bedtime have also been shown to blunt the nocturnal release of growth hormone.
RISK: 2 (moderate)
BENEFIT: 3 (high)

Not eating after training
Some popular fat loss programs specifically advise not eating for a specified period of time (usually one to two hours) after cardio (and or weight training) in order to "maximize the post-exercise fat burning effects of the cardio." While this may accelerate fat loss slightly, the risk of inadequate recovery and loss of

lean tissue is very high. The research is very clear on this point: There is a "window of opportunity" after training and the post workout meal (protein at the very least), should not be delayed, regardless of whether the activity is strength training or cardio training.

RISK: 3 (high)
BENEFIT: 1 (low)

CONCLUSION

The key to achieving optimal results seems to be risk management, rather than risk avoidance. An important point to realize is that high risk doesn't automatically mean that you will get injured or over trained. Kinakin said, "High risk only indicates the possibility, not the certainty of injury." Without the ability to make distinctions between risk and benefit, you may be missing out on much greater fat loss than you are capable of achieving. You may lose fat, but you might never achieve single digit body fat or extreme levels of leanness if that is your goal. All else being equal, the man or woman with the most choices and possibilities for action is the one who is most likely to succeed – not the person who always plays it safe.

About The Author

Tom Venuto is a lifetime natural bodybuilder, gym owner, freelance writer, success coach and author of the #1 best-selling e-book "Burn the Fat, Feed The Muscle" (BFFM). Tom has written over 160 articles and has been featured in IRONMAN magazine, Natural Bodybuilding, Muscular Development, Muscle-Zine, Exercise for Men and Men's Exercise. Tom's inspiring and informative articles on bodybuilding, weight loss and motivation are also featured regularly on dozens of websites worldwide. To subscribe to Tom's free monthly e-zine, visit the Fitness Renaissance website here: www.fitren.com

Hormone Modulation Therapy

The age-reversal premise outlined here is the subject of many books written by highly respected medical doctors. These books provide a persuasive compilation of research findings and clinical experience to document the safety and efficacy of using various approaches in treating ageing. The books fail, however, to provide an aggressive therapeutic plan of action. Here we have adapted the plan from The Life Extension Foundation. They provide a novel step-by-step program to enable people to immediately take advantage of this new information.

To understand the common mechanism, we first need to understand how aging itself occurs. To many, aging is simply a matter of wear and tear. Although often expressed in the scientific jargon of free radical damage to proteins and DNA or of reactive oxygen molecules and mitochondria, a simple homely model is often that of the aging car. Some scientists view getting old as the same thing that happens to a car, as it gathers rust, loses power, and falls apart. The problem with the car analogy is that organisms aren't cars. What car can continually repair itself for decades? If organisms were cars, then they would be remarkably wondrous cars with invisible, mechanisms that magically repair, replace, and tune up the car all the time. Imagine having a car in which every time a rust spot began to appear, the fender was magically replaced with a new one. Every time the tires lost a bit of their tread, the mechanism magically added more new rubber with deeper treads. Every time the spark plugs got dirty, the car would self tune, clean them, adjust the gaps or replace them. The oil was replaced every night, the paint redone every two days, the engine cleaned and tuned once a week. Magical, yes, but that is precisely what your body does all the time. You live in a body that actively resists wear and tear by continually repairing itself, replacing lost cells and damaged proteins, making new mitochondria and new molecules, fixing DNA and remaking itself from top to bottom. Quite some car.

And yet, this magical car, this body which continually repairs itself, grows old. The problem, however, lies not in the rust and the worn tread, but the fact that it stops repairing itself. There is always free radical damage, but older cells stop doing much about it. Every single one of your cells divided and ultimately came two joined cells, one from each of your parents (with the mitochondria from your mother), whose cells in turn came from their parents, and so on back as far as life has been around. Following your cells, (and their mitochondria) back through your maternal line, we quickly realize that you are part of a line of cells which are three and a half billion years old. You look pretty good, considering that free radical damage has been after your cells for several billion years. Why haven't *those* cells aged and died? Perhaps its not just free radical damage, but something about fertilization and having so many cells. But there are multicellular organisms that never age and single celled organisms that do. In fact, the reason that your cells age is that they *allow* themselves to do so.

Some cells, cancer cells or the germ cell lines that created you, never age. Other cells, such as most (though not all) of the cells of your body age, although at varying rates. All of these cells - aging or not, at different rates or not - are exposed to free radical and other damage, yet only certain cells age. The difference is that aging cells slow down their repair (and other) processes, while cells that don't age continue to deal with the damage, quite literally forever.

The following two segments deal with the hormone structure and requirements for adult men and women. How they change with age, and how the clock can literally be turned back. Following this segment we'll talk about (MVMS) multi vitamin mineral supplements. Without the proper vitamins and anti-oxidizing agents, our cells will prematurely oxidize and die.

Male Hormone Modulation Therapy

Female Hormone Modulation is after this section.

In writing this protocol, the Life Extension Foundation reviewed several thousand published scientific studies to validate safety and anti-aging efficacy. We also received input from experts who have personally followed this system for several years.

Foundation members do not want to see their bodies ravaged by age if a documented therapy is available that can control or reverse this devastating process. In this case, proven therapies exist and many of them are FDA approved.

Implementing this protocol requires diligent medical testing, but the potential for significant age reversal is compelling.

MALE HORMONES AND AGING

As men age past age 40, hormonal changes occur that slowly inhibit physical, sexual, and cognitive function. The outward appearance of a typical middle-aged male shows increased abdominal fat and shrinkage of muscle mass, a hallmark effect of hormone imbalance. Loss of a feeling of well-being, sometimes manifesting as depression, is a common psychological complication of hormone imbalance. Until recently, these changes were attributed to "growing old," and men were expected to accept the fact that their bodies were entering into a long degenerative process that would someday result in death.

A remarkable amount of data has been compiled indicating that many of the diseases that middle-aged men begin experiencing, including depression, fatigue, abdominal weight gain, alterations in mood and cognition, decreased libido, erectile dysfunction, prostate disease, and heart disease are directly related to hormone imbalances that are correctable with currently available drug and nutrient therapies. The onset of these symptoms usually appears in the early 50s, although with smokers the onset is significantly earlier.

To the patient's detriment, conventional doctors are increasingly prescribing drugs to treat depression, elevated cholesterol, angina, and a host of other diseases that might be caused by an underlying hormone imbalance.

If doctors checked their male patients' blood levels of estrogen, testosterone, thyroid, and DHEA (instead of prescribing drugs to treat symptoms), they might be surprised to learn that many problems could be eliminated by adjusting hormone levels to fit the profile of a healthy 21-year-old male.

Most physicians are not familiar with the hormone blood tests that should be ordered for men, nor do they have the experience required to properly adjust hormones to reverse the degenerative changes that begin in midlife. This protocol will provide the patient and physician with the information necessary to safely modulate hormone levels for the purpose of preventing and treating many of the common diseases associated with growing older.

Too Much Estrogen

The most significant hormone imbalance in aging men is a decrease in free testosterone, while estrogen levels remain the same or increase precipitously. As men grow older, they experience a variety of disorders relating to the dual effects of having too little testosterone and excess estrogen. The result is a testosterone-estrogen imbalance that directly causes many of the debilitating health problems associated with normal aging.

One cause of hormone imbalance in men is that their testosterone is increasingly converted to estrogen. One report showed that estrogen levels of the average 54-year-old man are higher than those of the average 59-year-old woman.

The reason that testosterone replacement therapy does not work by itself for many men is that exogenously administered testosterone may convert (aromatize) into even more estrogen, thus potentially worsening the hormone imbalance problem in aging males (i.e., too much estrogen and not enough free testosterone). Although there are studies that show that testosterone replacement therapy does not increase estrogen beyond normal reference ranges, we will show later how the standard laboratory reference ranges do not adequately address the issue of estrogen overload.

Estrogen is an essential hormone for men, but too much of it causes a wide range of health problems. The most dangerous acute effect of excess estrogen and too little testosterone is an increased risk of heart attack or stroke. High levels of estrogen have been implicated as a cause of benign prostatic hypertrophy (BPH). One mechanism by which nettle root extract works is to block the binding of growth-stimulating estrogen to prostate cells.

When there is too little testosterone present, estrogen attaches to testosterone cell receptor sites throughout the body and creates many problems in aging men. In youth, low amounts of estrogen are used to turn off the powerful cell-stimulating effects of testosterone. As estrogen levels increase with age, testosterone cell stimulation may be locked in the "off" position, thus reducing sexual arousal and sensation and causing the loss of libido so common in aging men.

High serum levels of estrogen also trick the brain into thinking that enough testosterone is being produced, further slowing the natural production of testosterone. This happens when estrogen saturates testosterone receptors in the hypothalamus region of the brain. The saturated hypothalamus then stops sending out a hormone to the pituitary gland to stimulate secretion of luteinizing hormone that the gonads require to produce testosterone. High estrogen can thus shut down the normal testicular production of testosterone.

One further complication of excess estrogen is that it increases the body's production of sex hormone-binding globulin (SHBG). SHBG binds free testosterone in the blood and makes it unavailable to cell receptor sites.

Based on the multiple deleterious effects of excess estrogen in men, aggressive action should be taken to reduce estrogen to a safe range if a blood test reveals elevated levels. We will discuss the appropriate blood tests and steps that can be taken to lower estrogen levels later in this protocol.

THE CRITICAL IMPORTANCE OF FREE TESTOSTERONE

Testosterone is much more than a sex hormone. There are testosterone receptor sites in cells throughout the body, most notably in the brain and heart. Youthful protein synthesis for maintaining muscle mass and bone formation requires testosterone. Testosterone improves oxygen uptake throughout the body, helps control blood sugar, regulates cholesterol, and maintains immune surveillance. The body requires testosterone to maintain youthful cardiac output and neurological function. Testosterone is also a critical hormone in the maintenance of healthy bone density, muscle mass, and red blood cell production.

Of critical concern to psychiatrists are studies showing that men with depression have lower levels of testosterone than do control subjects. For some men, elevating free testosterone levels could prove to be an effective antidepressant therapy. There is a basis for free testosterone levels being measured in men with depression and for replacement therapy being initiated if free testosterone levels are low normal or below normal.

Testosterone is one of the most misunderstood hormones. Body builders tarnished the reputation of testosterone by putting large amounts of synthetic testosterone drugs into their young bodies. Synthetic testosterone abuse can produce detrimental effects, but this has nothing to do with the benefits a man over age 40 can enjoy by properly restoring his natural testosterone to a youthful level.

Conventional doctors have not recommended testosterone replacement therapy because of an erroneous concern that testosterone causes prostate cancer. As we will later show, fear of prostate cancer is not a scientifically valid reason to avoid testosterone modulation therapy.

Another concern that skeptical physicians have about prescribing testosterone replacement therapy is that some poorly conducted studies showed it to be ineffective in the long-term treatment of aging. These studies indicate anti-aging benefits when testosterone is given, but the effects often wear off. What physicians fail to appreciate is that exogenously administered testosterone can convert to estrogen in the body. The higher estrogen levels may negate the benefits of the exogenously administered testosterone. The solution to the estrogen-overload problem is to block the conversion of testosterone to estrogen in the body.

Numerous studies show that maintaining youthful levels of free testosterone can enable the aging man to restore strength, stamina, cognition, heart function, sexuality, and outlook on life, that is, to alleviate depression. A study in Drugs and Aging (1999) suggested that androgen therapy can result in polycythemia (increased numbers of red blood cells) causing an increase in blood viscosity and risk of clotting. For many aging men, however, borderline anemia is a greater concern than red blood cell overproduction. When men are deprived of testosterone during prostate cancer therapy, anemia frequently manifests. Life Extension has not seen cases in which polycythemia developed in men taking enough testosterone to restore physiological youthful ranges. In other words, too much testosterone could cause problems, but replacing testosterone to that of a healthy 21-year-old should not produce the side effects that some doctors are unduly concerned about. As you will read in the section entitled "Testosterone and the Heart," it appears that testosterone replacement therapy provides significant beneficial effects against cardiovascular disease.

Why Testosterone Levels Decline

Testosterone production begins in the brain. When the hypothalamus detects a deficiency of testosterone in the blood, it secretes a hormone called gonadotrophin-releasing hormone to the pituitary gland. This prompts the pituitary to secrete luteinizing hormone (LH), which then prompts the Leydig cells in the testes to produce testosterone.

In some men, the testes lose their ability to produce testosterone, no matter how much LH is being produced. This type of testosterone deficiency is diagnosed when blood tests show high levels of LH and low levels of testosterone. In other words, the pituitary gland is telling the testes (by secreting LH) to produce testosterone, but the testes have lost their functional ability. So the pituitary gland vainly continues to secrete LH because there is not enough testosterone in the blood to provide a feedback mechanism that would tell the pituitary to shut down. In other cases, the hypothalamus, or pituitary gland, fails to produce sufficient amounts of LH, thus preventing healthy testes from secreting testosterone. Blood testing can determine whether sufficient amounts of LH are being secreted by the pituitary gland and help determine the appropriate therapeutic approach. If serum (blood) testosterone levels are very low, it is important to diagnose the cause, but no matter what the underlying problem, therapies exist today to safely restore testosterone to youthful levels in any man (who does not already have prostate cancer).

As indicated earlier, a major problem that aging men face is not low production of testosterone, but excessive conversion of testosterone to estrogen. Specific therapies to suppress excess estrogen and boost free testosterone back to youthful physiological levels will be discussed later.

The Effects of Testosterone on Libido

Sexual stimulation and erection begin in the brain when neuronal testosterone-receptor sites are prompted to ignite a cascade of biochemical events that involve testosterone-receptor sites in the nerves, blood vessels, and muscles. Free testosterone promotes sexual desire and then facilitates performance, sensation, and the ultimate degree of fulfillment.

Without adequate levels of free testosterone, the quality of a man's sex life is adversely affected and the genitals atrophy. When free testosterone is restored, positive changes can be expected in the structure and function of the sex organs. (It should be noted that sexual dysfunction can be caused by other factors unrelated to hormone imbalance. An example of such a factor is arteriosclerotic blockage of the penile arteries.)

The genital-pelvic region is packed with testosterone receptors that are ultra-sensitive to free testosterone-induced sexual stimulation. Clinical studies using testosterone injections, creams, or patches have often failed to provide a long-lasting, libido-enhancing effect in aging men. We now know why. The testosterone can be converted to estrogen. The estrogen is then taken up by testosterone receptor sites in cells throughout the body. When an estrogen molecule occupies a testosterone receptor site on a cell membrane, it blocks the ability of serum testosterone to induce a healthy hormonal signal. It does not matter how much serum free testosterone is available if excess estrogen is competing for the same cellular receptor sites.

Estrogen can also increase the production of SHBG, which binds the active free testosterone into an inactive "bound testosterone." Bound testosterone cannot be picked up by testosterone receptors on cell membranes. For testosterone to produce long-lasting, libido-enhancing effects, it must be kept in the "free" form (not bound to SHBG) in the bloodstream. It is also necessary to suppress excess estrogen because this hormone can compete for testosterone receptor sites in the sex centers of the brain and the genitals.

Restoring youthful hormone balance can have a significant impact on male sexuality.

Testosterone and the Heart

Normal aging results in the gradual weakening of the heart, even in the absence of significant coronary artery disease. If nothing else kills the elderly male, his heart just stops beating at some point.

Testosterone is a muscle-building hormone, and there are many testosterone-receptor sites in the heart. The weakening of the heart muscle can sometimes be attributed to testosterone deficiency.

Testosterone is not only responsible for maintaining heart muscle protein synthesis, it is also a promoter of coronary artery dilation and helps to maintain healthy cholesterol levels.

There are an ever-increasing number of studies indicating an association between high testosterone and low cardiovascular disease rates in men. In the majority of patients, symptoms and EKG measurements improve when low testosterone levels are corrected. One study showed that blood flow to the heart improved 68.8% in those receiving testosterone therapies. In China, doctors are successfully treating angina with testosterone therapy.

The following list represents the negative effects of low testosterone on cardiovascular disease:

- Cholesterol, fibrinogen, triglycerides, and insulin levels increase
- Coronary artery elasticity diminishes
- Blood pressure rises
- Human growth hormone (HGH) declines (weakening the heart muscle)
- Abdominal fat increases (increasing the risk of heart attack)

Those with cardiovascular disease should have their blood tested for free testosterone and estrogen. Some men (with full cooperation from their physicians) may be able to stop taking expensive drugs to stimulate cardiac output, lower cholesterol, and keep blood pressure under control if they correct a testosterone deficit or a testosterone-estrogen imbalance. A compelling study of 1100 men showed that those with serum dehydroepiandrosterone-sulfate (DHEA-S) in the lowest quarter (< 1.6 mcg/mL) were significantly more likely to incur symptoms of heart disease, and in a review of several studies, other authors have confirmed this association. Dehydroepiandro-sterone (DHEA) is produced by the adrenal gland and is a precursor hormone for the manufacture of testosterone.

Despite numerous studies substantiating the beneficial effects of testosterone therapy in treating heart disease, conventional cardiologists continue to overlook the important role this hormone plays in keeping their cardiac patients alive.

Testosterone and the Prostate Gland

Many doctors will tell you that testosterone causes prostate disease. The published scientific literature indicates otherwise.

As readers of Life Extension Magazine learned in late 1997, estrogen has been identified as a primary culprit in the development of benign prostatic hyperplasia (BPH). Estrogen has been shown to bind to SHBG in the prostate gland and cause the proliferation of epithelial cells in the prostate. This is corroborated by the fact that as men develop benign prostate enlargement, their levels of free testosterone plummet, although their estrogen levels remain the same or are rising. As previously discussed, aging men tend to convert their testosterone into estrogen. The published evidence shows that higher serum levels of testosterone are not a risk factor for developing benign prostate disease.

The major concern that has kept men from restoring their testosterone to youthful levels is the fear of prostate cancer. The theory is that since most prostate cancer cell lines need testosterone to proliferate, it is better not to replace the testosterone that is lost with aging. The problem with this theory is that most men who develop prostate cancer have low levels of testosterone, and the majority of published studies show that serum testosterone levels do not affect one's risk for contracting prostate cancer.

Because there is such a strong perception that any augmentation of testosterone can increase the risk of prostate cancer, we did a MEDLINE search on all the published studies relating to serum testosterone and prostate cancer. The abstracts at the end of this protocol provide quotations from the published literature as it relates to the issue of whether testosterone causes prostate disease. Of the 27 MEDLINE studies found, five studies indicated that men with higher testosterone levels had a greater incidence of prostate cancer, whereas 21 studies showed that testosterone was not a risk factor and one study was considered neutral. Before starting a testosterone replacement program, men should have a serum PSA test and a digital rectal exam to rule out prostate cancer. Nothing is risk free. A small minority of men with low testosterone and prostate cancer will not have an elevated PSA or palpable lesion detectable by digital rectal exam. If these men use supplemental testosterone, they risk an acute flare-up in their disease state. That is why PSA monitoring is so important every 30-45 days during the first 6 months of any type of testosterone augmentation therapy. If an underlying prostate cancer is detected because of testosterone therapy, it is usually treatable by no surgical means.

Please remember that testosterone does not cause acute prostate cancer, but if you have existing prostate cancer and do not know it, testosterone administration is likely to boost PSA sharply and provide your doctor with a quick diagnosis of prostate cancer (and an opportunity for very early treatment). We acknowledge that some aging men will not want to take this risk.

As stated above, the MEDLINE score was 21 to 5 against the theory that testosterone plays a role in the development of prostate cancer. None of these studies took into account the prostate cancer prevention effects for men who take lycopene, selenium, and vitamins A and E, nor did they factor in possible prostate disease preventives such as saw palmetto, nettle, soy, and pygeum.

In the book, *Maximize Your Vitality & Potency*, a persuasive case is made that testosterone and DHEA actually protect against the development of both benign and malignant prostate disease. Dr. Wright also points out that natural therapies, such as saw palmetto, nettle, and pygeum, provide a considerable degree of protection against the alleged negative effects that higher levels of testosterone might have on the prostate gland.

We eagerly await the results of more studies, but the fear of developing prostate cancer in the future should not be a reason to deprive your body today of the life-saving and life-enhancing benefits of restoring a youthful hormone balance.

Once a man has prostate cancer, testosterone therapy cannot be recommended because most prostate cancer cells use testosterone as a growth promoter. Regrettably, this denies prostate cancer patients the wonderful benefits of testosterone therapy. Men with severe BPH should approach testosterone replacement cautiously. It would be prudent for those with BPH who are taking testosterone replacement therapy to also use the drug Proscar (finasteride) to inhibit 5-alpha-reductase levels, thereby suppressing the formation of dihydrotestosterone (DHT). DHT is 10 times more potent than testosterone in promoting prostate growth, and suppressing DHT is a proven therapy in treating benign prostate enlargement. Saw palmetto extract suppresses some DHT in the prostate gland, but its effectiveness in alleviating symptoms of BPH probably has more to do with its blocking of alpha-adrenergic receptor sites on the sphincter muscle surrounding the urethra. (This is how the drug Hytrin works.)

Its inhibition of estrogen binding to prostate cells (such as nettle)

Its inhibition of the enzyme 3-ketosteroid (which causes the binding of DHT to prostate cells) Its anti-inflammatory effect on the prostate

Note: Men with severe BPH may also consider using the drug Arimidex (0.5 mg twice a week) to suppress excess levels of estrogen. Estrogen can worsen BPH and supplemental testosterone can elevate estrogen if an aromatase-inhibiting drug such as Arimidex is not used.

It is unfortunate that many people still think that restoring testosterone to youthful levels will increase the risk of prostate disease. This misconception has kept many men from availing themselves of this life-enhancing and life-saving hormone.

Although it is clear that excess estrogen causes benign prostate enlargement, the evidence for excess estrogen's role in the development of prostate cancer is uncertain. Some studies show that elevated estrogen is associated with increased prostate cancer risk, while other studies contradict this finding. For more information on testosterone, estrogen, and the prostate gland, refer to the February 1999 issue of Life Extension Magazine.

Testosterone and Depression

A consistent finding in the scientific literature is that testosterone replacement therapy produces an increased feeling of well-being. Published studies show that low testosterone correlates with symptoms of depression and other psychological disorders.

A common side effect of prescription antidepressant drugs is the suppression of libido. Those with depression either accept this drug-induced reduction in quality of life, or get off the antidepressant drugs so they can at least have a somewhat normal sex life. If more psychiatrists tested their patients' blood for free testosterone and prescribed natural testosterone therapies to those with low free testosterone, the need for libido-suppressing antidepressant drugs could be reduced or eliminated. As previously described, testosterone replacement often enhances libido, the opposite effect of most prescription antidepressants.

One study showed that patients with major depression experienced improvement that was equal to that achieved with standard antidepressant drugs.

Androderm is one of several natural testosterone-replacement therapies that can be prescribed by doctors. A 12-month clinical trial using this FDA-approved drug resulted in a statistically significant reduction in the depression score (6.9 before versus 3.9 after). Also noted were highly significant decreases in fatigue: from 79% before the patch to only 10% after 12 months.

According to Jonathan Wright, M.D., co-author of Maximize Your Vitality & Potency, the following effects have been reported in response to low testosterone levels:

- Loss of ability to concentrate
- Moodiness and emotionality
- Touchiness and irritability
- Great timidity
- Feeling weak
- Inner unrest
- Memory failure
- Reduced intellectual agility
- Passive attitudes
- General tiredness
- Reduced interest in surroundings
- Hypochondria

The above feelings can all be clinical symptoms of depression, and testosterone replacement therapy has been shown to alleviate these conditions. Testosterone thus has exciting therapeutic potential in the treatment of depression in men.

Testosterone and Mental Decline

Evidence indicates that low levels of testosterone may contribute to memory impairment and increase the vulnerability of the brain to Alzheimer's and related disorders. Beta-amyloid, a peptide that may accumulate in certain regions of the aging brain, is implicated in the development of Alzheimer's disease. Researchers have found that testosterone exerts neuroprotective benefits from the effects of toxic beta-amyloid. An article published in Brain Research describes a study in which cultured neurons were exposed to beta-amyloid in the presence of testosterone. The resulting toxicity from beta-amyloid was significantly reduced by testosterone through a rapid estrogen-independent mechanism.

Other researchers have explored the mechanism by which testosterone may exert its protective effect in Alzheimer's disease. Their research in animals shows that testosterone decreases the secretion of harmful beta-amyloid and increases the secretion of the non-amyloidogenic APP fragment, sbetaAPPalpha, indicating that testosterone supplementation in elderly men may be beneficial in the treatment of Alzheimer's.

Another published study examined the neuroprotective effects of estradiol, testosterone, epi-testosterone, and methyl-testosterone in neurons induced to undergo apoptosis by serum deprivation. Physiologic concentrations of testosterone were found to be neuroprotective, similar to estradiol. Methyl-testosterone showed an effect that was delayed in time, suggesting that a metabolite may be the active agent. Epi-testosterone showed a slight neuroprotective effect but not through the androgen receptor. The authors concluded that androgens may be of therapeutic value against Alzheimer's disease in aging males.

Researchers in Oxford, England found that lower levels of testosterone were present in men with Alzheimer's as opposed to controls. These results were independent of confounding factors such as age, body mass index, education, smoking, alcohol abuse, and endocrine therapy. The authors recommended further studies to determine whether low levels of total testosterone precede or follow the onset of Alzheimer's disease.

Testosterone and Aging

We know that many of the degenerative diseases of aging in men, such as Type-II diabetes, osteoporosis, and cardiovascular disease, are related to a testosterone deficiency. We also know that common characteristics of middle age and older age, such as depression, abdominal fat deposition, muscle atrophy, low energy, and cognitive decline, are also associated with less than optimal levels of free testosterone.

A consistent pattern that deals with fundamental aging shows that low testosterone causes excess production of a dangerous hormone called cortisol. Some anti-aging experts call cortisol a "death hormone" because of the multiple degenerative effects that it produces. Some of these effects are immune dysfunction, brain cell injury, and arterial wall damage.

A group of scientists conducted two double-blind studies in which they administered supplemental testosterone to groups of aging men and observed the typical responses of lower levels of cholesterol, glucose, and triglycerides, reductions in blood pressure, and decreased abdominal fat mass. The scientists showed that excess cortisol suppressed testosterone and growth hormone production and that the administration of testosterone acted as a "shield" against the overproduction of cortisol in the adrenal gland. Another study published in 1999 on testosterone and atherosclerosis in men showed a statistically significant correlation between low testosterone and excess serum insulin. It was noted that an elevated estradiol to testosterone ratio is connected with insulin resistance.

It is important to point out that testosterone is an anabolic (or protein building) hormone while cortisol is a catabolic hormone that breaks down proteins in the body. Normal aging consists of a progressive decrease in free testosterone with a marked increase in cortisol. As men age past 40, cortisol begins to dominate, and the catabolic effects associated with growing older begin to dominate.

These findings have significant implications in the battle to maintain youthful hormone balance for the purpose of staving off normal aging and its associated degenerative diseases.

THE TESTOSTERONE DOCTOR

Eugene Shippen, M.D. (co-author of The Testosterone Syndrome, 1998) provided extensive evidence documenting the pathology of the testosterone deficiency syndrome in men. Some excerpts follow from a lecture presented by Dr. Shippen at the American Academy for Anti-Aging Medicine Conference in December 1998:

First, testosterone is not just a "sex hormone." It should be seen as a "total body hormone," affecting every cell in the body. The changes seen in aging, such as the loss of lean body mass, the decline in energy, strength, and stamina, unexplained depression, and decrease in sexual sensation and performance, are all directly related to testosterone deficiency. Degenerative diseases such as heart disease, stroke, diabetes, arthritis, osteoporosis, and hypertension are all directly or indirectly linked to testosterone decline. Secondly, testosterone also functions as a pro-hormone. Local tissue conversion to estrogens, dihydrotestosterone (DHT), or other active metabolites plays an important part in cellular physiology.

Excess estrogen seems to be the culprit in prostate enlargement. Low testosterone levels are in fact associated with more aggressive prostate cancer. While fear of prostate cancer keeps many men from testosterone replacement, it is in fact testosterone deficiency that leads to the pathology that favors the development of prostate cancer.

Testosterone improves cellular bioenergetics. It acts as a cellular energizer. Since testosterone increases the metabolic rate and aerobic metabolism, it also dramatically improves glucose metabolism and lowers insulin resistance.

Another myth is that testosterone is bad for the heart. Actually, low testosterone correlates with heart disease more reliably than does high cholesterol. Testosterone is the most powerful cardiovascular protector for men. Testosterone strengthens the heart muscle; there are more testosterone receptors in the heart than in any other muscle. Testosterone lowers LDL cholesterol and total cholesterol and improves every cardiac risk factor. It has been shown to improve or eliminate arrhythmia and angina. Testosterone replacement is the most underutilized important treatment for heart disease.

Testosterone shines as a blood thinner, preventing blood clots.
Testosterone also helps prevent colon cancer.

Previous research on testosterone used the wrong form of replacement. Injections result in initial excess of testosterone, with conversion of excess to estrogens. Likewise, total testosterone is often measured instead of free testosterone, the bioavailable form. Some studies do not last long enough to show improvement. For instance, it may take six months to a year before the genital tissue fully recovers from atrophy caused by testosterone deficiency, and potency is restored.

Physicians urgently need to be educated about the benefits of testosterone and the delicate balance between androgens (testosterone) and estrogens. Each individual has his or her own pattern of hormone balance; this indicates that hormone replacement should be individualized and carefully monitored.

OBESITY AND HORMONE IMBALANCE

A consistent finding in the scientific literature is that obese men have low testosterone and very high estrogen levels. Central or visceral obesity ("pot belly") is recognized as a risk factor for cardiovascular disease and Type-II diabetes. Research has shed light on subtle hormone imbalances of borderline character in obese men that often fall within the normal laboratory reference range. Boosting testosterone levels seems to decrease the abdominal fat mass, reverse glucose intolerance, and reduce lipoprotein abnormalities in the serum. Further analysis has also disclosed a regulatory role for testosterone in counteracting visceral fat accumulation. Epidemiological data demonstrate that relatively low testosterone levels are a risk factor for development of visceral obesity.

One study showed that serum estrone and estradiol were elevated twofold in one group of morbidly obese men. Fat cells synthesize the aromatase enzyme, causing male hormones to convert to estrogens. Fat tissues, especially in the abdomen, have been shown to literally "aromatize" testosterone and its precursor hormones into potent estrogens.

Eating high-fat foods may reduce free testosterone levels according to one study that measured serum levels of sex steroid hormones after ingestion of different types of food. High-protein and high-carbohydrate meals had no effect on serum hormone levels, but a fat-containing meal reduced free testosterone levels for 4 hours.

Obese men have testosterone deficiency caused by the production of excess aromatase enzyme in fat cells and also from the fat they consume in their diet. The resulting hormone imbalance (too much estrogen and not enough free testosterone) in obese men partially explains why so many are impotent and have a wide range of premature degenerative diseases.

FACTORS CAUSING THE ESTROGEN-TESTOSTERONE IMBALANCE IN MEN

If your blood tests reveal high estrogen and low testosterone, here are the common factors involved:

Excess "Aromatase" Enzyme

As men age, they produce larger quantities of an enzyme called aromatase. The aromatase enzyme converts testosterone into estrogen in the body. Inhibiting the aromatase enzyme results in a significant decline in estrogen levels while often boosting free testosterone to youthful levels. Therefore, an agent designated as an "aromatase inhibitor" may be of special value to aging men who have excess estrogen.

Liver Enzymatic Activity

A healthy liver eliminates surplus estrogen and sex hormone-binding globulin. Aging, alcohol, and certain drugs impair liver function and can be a major cause of hormone imbalance in aging men. Heavy alcohol intake increases estrogen in men and women.

Obesity

Fat cells create aromatase enzyme and especially contribute to the buildup of abdominal fat. Low testosterone allows the formation of abdominal fat, which then causes more aromatase enzyme formation and thus even lower levels of testosterone and higher estrogen (by aromatizing testosterone into estrogen). It is especially important for overweight men to consider hormone modulation therapy.

Zinc Deficiency

Zinc is a natural aromatase enzyme inhibitor. Since most Life Extension Foundation members consume adequate amounts of zinc (30-90 mg a day), elevated estrogen in Foundation members is often caused by factors other than zinc deficiency.

Lifestyle Changes

Lifestyle changes (such as reducing alcohol intake) can produce a dramatic improvement in the estrogen-testosterone balance, but many people need to use aromatase-inhibiting agents to lower estrogen and to improve their liver function to remove excess SHBG. Aromatase converts testosterone into estrogen and can indirectly increase SHBG. SHBG binds to free testosterone and prevents it from exerting its biochemical effects in the body.

CORRECTING A HORMONE IMBALANCE

A male hormone imbalance can be detected through use of the proper blood tests and can be corrected using available drugs and nutrients. The following represents a step-by-step program to safely restore youthful hormone balance in aging men:

Step 1: Blood Testing

The following initial blood tests are recommended for men over age 40:

- Complete blood count and chemistry profile to include liver-kidney function, glucose, minerals, lipids, and thyroid (TSH)
- Free and Total Testosterone
- Estradiol (estrogen)
- DHT (dihydrotestosterone)
- DHEA
- PSA
- Homocysteine
- Luteinizing hormone (LH) (optional)
- Sex Hormone Binding Globulin (SHBG) (optional)

Step 2: Interpretation of Free Testosterone,

Estrogen, and Total Testosterone Blood Test Results

One can easily determine if they need testosterone replacement or estrogen suppression by adhering to the following guidelines:

Free Testosterone

Free testosterone blood levels should be at the high-normal of the reference range. We define high-normal range as the upper one third of the reference range. Under no circumstances should free or total testosterone be above the high end of the normal range.

What too often happens is that a standard laboratory "reference range" deceives a man (and his physician) into believing that proper hormone balance exists because the results of a free testosterone test fall within the "normal" range. The following charts show a wide range of so-called "normal" ranges of testosterone for men of various ages. While these normal ranges may reflect population "averages," the objective for most men over age 40 is to be in the upper one-third testosterone range of the 21- to 29-year-old group. Based on the following reference range chart from LabCorp, this means that optimal free testosterone levels should be between 21-26.5 nanogram/dL in aging men.

Reference Intervals for Free Testosterone from LabCorp

- 20-29 years 9.3-26.5 picogram/mL
- 30-39 years 8.7-25.1 picogram/mL
- 40-49 years 6.8-21.5 picogram/mL
- 50-59 years 7.2-24.0 picogram/mL
- 60+ years 6.6-18.1 picogram/mL

An example of how this chart can be deceptive would be if a 50-year-old man presented symptoms of testosterone deficiency (depression, low energy, abdominal obesity, angina, etc.), but his blood test revealed his free testosterone to be 9 picogram/mL. His doctor might tell him he is fine because he falls within the normal "reference range." The reality may be that to achieve optimal benefits, testosterone levels should be between 21-26.5 picogram/mL. That means a man could have less than half the amount of testosterone needed to overcome symptoms of a testosterone deficiency, but his doctor will not prescribe testosterone replacement because the man falls within the "average" parameters. That is why it is so important to differentiate between "average" and "optimal." Average 50-year-old men often have the symptoms of having too little testosterone. Yet since so many 50-year-old men have lower than desired testosterone levels, this is considered to be "normal" when it comes to standard laboratory reference ranges.

The Life Extension Foundation would like to point out that there is disagreement between clinicians and laboratories on the best method for measuring testosterone status. There are different schools of thought as to which form of testosterone should be measured and which analytical procedure provides the most accurate assessment of metabolic activity.

To illustrate this point, the reference values for measuring free testosterone from Quest Diagnostics follow:

Adult Male (20-60+ years):

- 1.0-2.7%   50-210 pg/mL
- Optimal Range: 150-210 pg/mL
  (for aging men without prostate cancer)

We believe that direct testing for free testosterone is the best way to test for testosterone activity, as free testosterone is active testosterone and consists of only 1-2% of total testosterone. Total testosterone can be good for general testing. The four main methods presently used for analyzing free testosterone are:

1. Direct, Free Testosterone by
   Direct Analog/Radioimmunoassay (RIA)
2. Testosterone Free by Ultrafiltration (UF)
3. Testosterone Free by Equilibrium Tracer Dialysis (ETD)
4. Testosterone Free and Weakly Bound by Radioasssay (FWRA)

The latter three test methods are older, more complicated methods that are technically demanding. The direct RIA test has a number of commercial test kits available, and they are better used in today's automated equipment, making this test less tedious and requiring a smaller (less) sample. These advantages have convinced many laboratories and clinics to prefer direct RIA testing for free testosterone. The Life Extension Foundation agrees with this assessment, and therefore uses and recommends the direct free testosterone test with the above-mentioned reference levels.

Consequently, if your doctor tests your free testosterone, be sure you know the analytical method used. If your test results have a reference range as follows, you have probably been tested with one of the other test methods:

Test Type	Male Reference Range
FWRA	66-417 nanogram/dL
%FWRA	12.3-63%
UF or ETD	5-21 nanogram/dL
UF or ETD	50-210 picogram/mL
% of free by UF or ETD	1.0-2.7%

No matter what test method is used to determine your free testosterone status, the optimal level (where you want to be) is in the upper one-third of normal for a 20-29 year old male.

Estrogen

Estrogen (measured as estradiol) should be in the mid- to lower-normal range. If estradiol levels are in the upper one-third of the normal reference range, or above the normal reference range, this excessive level of estrogen should be reduced. Labcorp lists a reference range of between 3-70 picogram/mL for estradiol while Quest states a reference range of between 10-50. For optimal health, estradiol should be in the range of **10-30** picogram/mL for a man of any age.

The fact that most aging men have too much estrogen does not mean it is acceptable for a man to have low estrogen. Estrogen is used by men to maintain bone density, and abnormally low estrogen levels may increase the risk for prostate cancer and osteoporosis. The objective is to achieve hormone balance, not to create sky-high testosterone levels without enough estrogen. The problem is that, if we do nothing, most men will have too much estrogen and far too little testosterone.

Total Testosterone

Some men have their total testosterone measured. Standard reference ranges are between 241-827 nanograms/dL for most laboratories. Many older men are below 241. Optimal levels of total testosterone for most men are between 500-827 nanograms/dL. If your levels are lower than 500 nanograms/dL or even a little higher and you still have symptoms, you should check your free testosterone by the Direct (RIA) method.

For other hormone tests, the following are considered to be optimal:

Where You Want to Be

PSA Under 2.6 ng/mL (optimal range)
Standard reference range is up to 4, but if your level is persistently 2.6 or above, have a blood test to measure the percentage of free vs. bound PSA and a digital rectal exam to help rule out prostate cancer.

DHEA 400-560 mcg/dL (optimal range)
For older men, standard DHEA ranges are very low. It is important for men without prostate cancer to restore them to the youthful range (400-560).

DHT 20-50 nanogram/dL (optimal range)
Reference range is 30-85. DHT is 10 times more androgenic than testosterone and has been implicated in prostate problems and hair loss.

Luteinizing hormone (LH) Under 9.3 mIU/mL (optimal range)
Standard reference ranges are base on age:
Age
20-70: 1.5-9.3 mIU/mL
70+: 3.1-34.6 mIU/mL

If these levels are high, it is an indication of testicular testosterone production deficiency. LH tells the testes to produce testosterone. If there is too little testosterone present, the pituitary gland secretes more LH in a futile effort to stimulate testicular testosterone production. Testosterone replacement therapy should suppress excess LH levels. Low LH can also be a sign of estrogen overload, since too much estrogen can suppress LH activity. This could mean using an estrogen blocker like Arimidex could solve a testosterone deficiency problem.

Sex Hormone Binding Under 30 nanomoles/L (optimal range)
Reference range is 13-71 nanomole/L. Excessive binding inactivates testosterone.

There are five possible reasons why free testosterone levels may be low-normal (below the upper third of the highest number of the reference range):

1. Too much testosterone is being converted to estradiol by excess aromatase enzyme and/or the liver is failing to adequately detoxify surplus estrogen. Excess aromatase enzyme and/or liver dysfunction is likely the cause if estradiol levels are over 30. Remember, aromatase converts testosterone into estradiol, which can cause estrogen overload and testosterone deficiency.

111

2. Too much free testosterone is being bound by SHBG (sex hormone binding globulin). This would be especially apparent if total testosterone levels were in the high normal range, while free testosterone was below the upper one-third range.

3. The pituitary gland fails to secrete adequate amounts of luteinizing hormone (LH) to stimulate testicular production of testosterone. Total testosterone in this case would be in the bottom one-third to one-half range. (On LabCorp's scale, this would be a number below 241-500 ng/dL.)

4. The testes have lost their ability to produce testosterone, despite adequate amounts of the testicular-stimulating luteinizing hormone. In this case, LH would be above normal, and total testosterone would in very low normal or below normal ranges.

5. Inadequate amounts of DHEA are being produced in the body. (DHEA is a precursor hormone to testosterone and estrogen).

Step 3: What to Do When Results Are Less Than Optimal

If estradiol levels are high (above 30), total testosterone is mid to high-normal, and free testosterone levels are low or low-normal (at the bottom one third of the highest number on the reference range), you should:

Make sure you are getting 80 mg a day of zinc. (Zinc functions as an aromatase inhibitor for some men.)

Consume 400 mg of indole-3-carbinol to help neutralize dangerous estrogen metabolites. Cruciferous vegetables, such as broccoli and cauliflower, can also stimulate the liver to metabolize and excrete excess estrogen.

Reduce or eliminate alcohol consumption to enable your liver to better remove excess estrogens.

Review all drugs you are regularly taking to see if they may be interfering with healthy liver function. Common drugs that affect liver function are the NSAIDs: ibuprofen, acetaminophen, aspirin, the "statin" class of cholesterol-lowering drugs, some heart and blood pressure medications, and some antidepressants. It is interesting to note that drugs being prescribed to treat the symptoms of testosterone deficiency such as the statins and certain antidepressants may actually aggravate a testosterone deficit, thus making the cholesterol problem or depression worse.

Lose weight. Fat cells, especially in the abdominal region, produce the aromatase enzyme, which converts testosterone into estrogen.

Take a combination supplement providing a flavonoid called chrysin (1000 mg) along with piperine (10 mg) to enable the chrysin to be absorbed into the blood stream. Chrysin has been shown to be a mild aromatase inhibitor. This combination of chrysin and peperine can be found in a product called Super MiraForte.

If all of the above fail to increase free testosterone and lower excess estradiol, ask your doctor to prescribe the potent aromatase inhibiting drug Arimidex (anastrozole) in the very low dose of 0.5 mg twice a week. Arimidex is prescribed to breast cancer patients at the dose of 1-10 mg a day. Even at the higher dose prescribed to cancer patients, side effects are rare. In the minute dose of 0.5 mg twice a week, a man will see an immediate drop in estradiol levels and should experience a rise in free testosterone to the optimal range.

If free testosterone levels are in the lower two thirds of the highest number in the reference range, but total testosterone is high-normal, and estradiol levels are not over 30, you should:

Consider following some of the recommendations in the previous section to inhibit aromatase because many of the same factors are involved in excess SHBG activity.

Take 320 mg a day of the super-critical extract of saw palmetto and 240 mg a day of the methanolic extract of nettle (Urtica dioica). Nettle may specifically inhibit SHGB, while saw palmetto may reduce the effects of excess estrogen by blocking the nuclear estrogen receptor sites in prostate cells, which in turn activate the cell-stimulating effects of testosterone and dihydrotestosterone. Saw palmetto also has the effect of blocking the oxidation of testosterone to androstenedione, a potent androgen that has been implicated in the development of prostate disease.

If total testosterone is in the lower third of the reference range or below normal, and free testosterone is low, and estradiol levels are under 30, you should

Initiate therapy with the testosterone patch, pellet, or cream. Do not use testosterone injections or tablets.

OR

See if your luteinizing hormone (LH) is below normal. If LH is low, your doctor can prescribe an individual dose of chorionic gonadotropin (HCG) hormone for injection. Chorionic gonadotropic hormone functions similarly to LH and can re-start testicular production of testosterone. Your doctor can instruct you about how to use tiny 30-gauge needles to give yourself injections 2-3 times a week.

After 1 month on chorionic gonadotropic hormone, a blood test can determine whether total testosterone levels are significantly increasing. You may also see your testicles growing larger.

Before initiating testosterone replacement therapy, have a PSA blood test and a digital rectal exam to rule out detectable prostate cancer. Once total testosterone levels are restored to a high-normal range, monitor blood levels of estradiol, free testosterone, and PSA every 30-45 days for the first 6 months to make sure the exogenous testosterone you are using is following a healthy metabolic pathway and not causing a flare-up of an underlying prostate cancer. The objective is to raise your levels of free testosterone to the upper third of the reference range, but to not increase estradiol levels beyond 30.

Excess estrogen (estradiol) blocks the production and effect of testosterone throughout the body, dampens sexuality, and increases the risk of prostate and cardiovascular disease. Once you have established the proper ratio of free testosterone (upper third of the highest number in the reference range) and estradiol (not more than 30), make sure your blood is tested every 30-45 days for the first 5 months. Test every 6 months thereafter for free testosterone, estradiol, and PSA. For men in their 40s-50s, correcting the excess level of estradiol is often all that has to be done.

THERAPIES

"Andro" Supplements

Androstenedione is a precursor to both testosterone and estrogen. Early studies showed that "andro" supplements could markedly increase testosterone levels, but more recent studies cast doubt on this concept. A study in the Journal of the American Medical Association (1999) reported on an 8-week study showing that androstenedione supplements increased estrogen levels in 30 men. No increase in strength, muscle mass, or testosterone levels was observed. Perhaps combining androstenedione with an aromatase inhibitor that would prevent it from converting to estrogen would make this precursor hormone work better in men. In the meantime, we suggest avoiding androstenedione until more definitive research is published.

Testosterone Patches, Creams, Pellets, and Tablets

Synthetic testosterone "steroid" drugs are chemically different from the testosterone your body makes and do not provide the same effect as natural testosterone. Some of the synthetic testosterone drugs to avoid using on a long-term basis are methyltestosterone, danazol, oxandrolone, testosterone propionate, cypionate, or enanthate.

The fact that testosterone is marketed as a "drug" does not mean it is not the same natural hormone your body produced. Scientists learned decades ago how to make the identical testosterone that your body produces, but since natural testosterone could not be patented, drug companies developed all kinds of synthetic testosterone analogs that could be patented and approved by the FDA as new drugs. Currently available recommended natural testosterone drugs are:

- Androderm Transdermal System (SmithKline Beecham's testosterone patch)
- Testoderm Transdermal System (Alza's testosterone patch)
- Testosterone creams, pellets, and sublingual tablets (available from compounding pharmacies)

Both synthetic and natural testosterone drugs require a prescription, and a prescription should only be written after blood or saliva tests reveal a testosterone deficiency.

Alternative physicians usually prescribe testosterone creams and other types made at compounding pharmacies, whereas conventional doctors are more likely to prescribe a box of ready-made, FDA-approved testosterone patches. All forms of natural testosterone are the same and all will markedly increase free testosterone in the blood or saliva.

If you interact with children, you may want to avoid testosterone creams. There is a report of a young male child going through premature puberty after the child made contact with the testosterone cream on his father's body and on weightlifting equipment in the home. This unique case is a testament to the powerful effects that testosterone exerts in the body.

Caution: Do not use testosterone replacement if you have prostate cancer.

Men with existing prostate cancer should follow an opposite approach as it relates to testosterone. Prostate cancer patients are normally prescribed testosterone ablation therapy (using a drug that blocks the pituitary release of LH and another drug that blocks testosterone-receptor sites on the cells). Early-stage prostate cancer cells can often be controlled by totally suppressing testosterone in the body. Late-stage prostate cancer patients are sometimes put on drugs that produce estrogenic effects to suppress prostate cancer cells that no longer depend on testosterone for growth. Regrettably, prostate cancer patients on testosterone ablation therapy often temporarily have many of the unpleasant effects of low testosterone that have been described in this article. Before initiating a therapy that boosts your free testosterone level, a blood PSA test and digital rectal exam are recommended for men over age 40. While restoring free testosterone to healthy physiological levels does not cause prostate cancer, it can induce existing prostate cancer cells to proliferate faster.

Natural Testosterone-Boosting/Estrogen-Suppressing Approaches

Chrysin

A bioflavonoid called chrysin has shown potential as a natural aromatase-inhibitor. Chrysin can be extracted from various plants. Bodybuilders have used it as a testosterone-boosting supplement because by inhibiting the aromatase enzyme, less testosterone is converted into estrogen. The problem with chrysin is that because of its poor absorption into the bloodstream, it has not produced the testosterone-enhancing effects users expect.

In a study published in Biochemical Pharmacology (1999), the specific mechanisms of chrysin's absorption impairment were identified, which infers that the addition of a pepper extract (piperine) could significantly enhance the bioavailability of chrysin. Pilot studies have found that when chrysin is combined with piperine, reductions in serum estrogen (estradiol) and increases in total and free testosterone result in 30 days. Aromatase-inhibiting drugs are used to treat women with estrogen-dependent breast cancers. The rationale for this therapy is that estrogen is produced by fat cells via a process known as aromatization. Aging men often have excess aromatase enzyme activity, and the result is that too much of their testosterone is "aromatized" into estrogen.

In a study published in the Journal of Steroid Biochemical Molecular Biology (1993), chrysin and 10 other flavonoids were compared to an aromatase-inhibiting drug (aminoglutethimide). The study tested the aromatase-inhibiting effects of these natural flavonoids (such as genistein, rutin, tea catechins, etc.) in human fat cell cultures. Chrysin was the most potent aromatase-inhibitor, and was shown to be similar in potency and effectiveness to the aromatase-inhibiting drug. The scientists conducting the study concluded by stating that the aromatase-inhibiting effects of certain flavonoids may contribute to the cancer preventive effects of plant-based diets.

116

Two studies have identified specific mechanisms by which chrysin inhibits aromatase in human cells. These studies demonstrate that chrysin is a more potent inhibitor of the aromatase enzyme than phytoestrogens and other flavonoids that are known to have aromatase-inhibiting properties. The purpose of these studies was to ascertain which fruits and vegetables should be included in the diet of postmenopausal women to reduce the incidence of breast cancer. Excess levels of mutagenic forms of estrogen have been linked to a greater risk of breast cancer, and scientists are studying dietary means of naturally reducing levels of these dangerous estrogens. Flavonoids such as chrysin are of considerable interest because they suppress excess estrogen via their aromatase-inhibiting properties. Although this cancer preventing effect is most important for women, inhibiting aromatase in aging men has tremendous potential for naturally suppressing excess estrogen while boosting low levels of testosterone to a youthful state.

Since chrysin is not a patentable drug, do not expect to see a lot of human research documenting its effects. There are many FDA-approved drugs that inhibit aromatase (such as Arimidex), and there is not much economic interest in finding natural ways of replacing these drugs. Although prescription aromatase-inhibiting drugs are relatively free of side effects, aging men who are seeking to gain control over their sex hormone levels sometimes prefer natural sources, rather than trying to convince a physician to prescribe a drug (such as Arimidex) that is not yet approved by the FDA as an antiaging therapy. (Arimidex is prescribed to estrogen-dependant breast cancer patients to prevent testosterone and other hormones in the body from converting, i.e., aromatasing, into estrogen.)

An advantage to using plant extracts to boost testosterone in lieu of drugs is that the plant extracts have ancillary health benefits. Chrysin, for example, is a potent antioxidant that produces vitamin-like effects in the body. It has been shown to induce an anti-inflammatory effect, possibly through inhibition of the enzymes 5-lipooxygenase and cyclooxygenase inflammation pathways. Aging is being increasingly viewed as a proinflammatory process, and agents that inhibit chronic inflammation may protect against diseases as diverse as atherosclerosis, senility, and aortic valve stenosis. Chrysin is one of many flavonoids being studied as a phyto-extract that may prevent some forms of cancer. If chrysin can boost free testosterone in the aging male by inhibiting the aromatase enzyme, this would provide men with a low-cost natural supplement that could provide the dual antiaging benefits of testosterone replacement and aromatase-inhibiting drug therapy. Pilot studies indicate that chrysin increases total and free testosterone levels in the majority of men who take it with piperine.

117

Chrysin has one other property that could add to its libido-enhancing potential. A major cause of sexual dissatisfaction among men is work-related stress and anxiety. Another problem some men have is "sexual performance anxiety" that prevents them from being able to achieve erections when they are expected to. In a study published in Pharmacology Biochemistry and Behavior (1994), mice were injected with diazepam (Valium), chrysin, or placebo to evaluate the effects these substances had on anxiety and performance levels. Chrysin was shown to produce antianxiety effects comparable with diazepam, but without sedation and muscle relaxation. In other words, chrysin produced a relaxing effect in the brain, but with no impairment of motor activity. The mechanism of action of chrysin was compared to diazepam, and it was shown that unlike diazepam, chrysin can reduce anxiety without inducing the common side effects associated with benzodiazepine drugs.

A common problem with benzodiazepine drugs is memory impairment. In a study published in Pharmacology Biochemistry and Behavior (1997), chrysin displayed potent antianxiety effects in rats, but did not interfere with cognitive performance. In this study, diazepam was shown to inhibit neurological function, but chrysin (and other antianxiety flavonoids) had no effect on training or test session performance. The scientists conducting this study pointed out that chrysin selectively inhibits anxiety in the brain but, unlike diazepam, does not induce the cognitive impairment.

Chrysin may therefore offer libido-enhancing effects in the aging male by:

Increasing free testosterone

Decreasing excess estrogen

Producing a safe antianxiety effect

Chrysin is being sold to bodybuilders by commercial supplement companies that do not know if their product is favorably modulating testosterone and estrogen levels in men. The Life Extension Foundation, on the other hand, has conducted studies to evaluate the effects of chrysin (combined with piperine to facilitate absorption) on aging men.

Nettle

About 90% of testosterone is produced by the testes; the remainder is produced by the adrenal glands. Testosterone functions as an aphrodisiac hormone in brain cells and as an anabolic hormone in the development of bone and skeletal muscle. But testosterone that becomes bound to serum globulin is not available to cell receptor sites and fails to induce a libido effect. It is therefore desirable to increase levels of "free testosterone" in order to ignite sexual arousal in the brain.

As discussed already, a hormone that controls levels of free testosterone is called SHBG. When testosterone binds to SHBG, it loses its biological activity and becomes known as "bound testosterone," as opposed to the desirable "free testosterone." As men age past age 45, SHBG's binding capacity increases almost dramatically--by 40% on average--and coincides with the age-associated loss of libido.

Some studies show that the decline in sexual interest with advancing age is not always due to the amount of testosterone produced, but rather to the increased binding of testosterone to globulin by SHBG. This explains why some older men who are on testosterone replacement therapy do not report a long-term aphrodisiac effect. That is, the artificially administered testosterone becomes bound by SHBG and is not bioavailable to cellular receptor sites where it would normally produce a libido-enhancing effect.

It should be noted that the liver also causes testosterone to bind to globulin. This liver-induced binding of testosterone is worsened by the use of sedatives, antihypertensives, tranquilizers, and alcoholic beverages. The overuse of drugs and alcohol could explain why some men do not experience a libido-enhancing effect when consuming drugs and plant-based aphrodisiacs. An interesting review entitled "How Desire Dies" discusses how frequently prescribed drugs, such as beta-blockers and antidepressants, cause sexual dysfunction. Prescription drugs of all types have been linked to inhibition of libido.

Logically, one way of increasing libido in older men would be to block the testosterone-binding effects of SHBG. This would leave more testosterone in its free, sexually activating form.

A highly concentrated extract from the nettle root provides a unique mechanism for increasing levels of free testosterone. European research has identified constituents of nettle root that bind to SHBG in place of testosterone, thus reducing SHBG's binding of free testosterone. As the authors of one study stated, these constituents of nettle root "may influence the blood level of free, i.e., active, steroid hormones by displacing them from the SHBG binding site."

The prostate gland also benefits from nettle root. In Germany, nettle root has been used as a treatment for benign prostatic hyperplasia (enlargement of the prostate gland) for decades. A metabolite of testosterone called dihydrotestosterone (DHT) stimulates prostate growth, leading to enlargement. Nettle root inhibits the binding of DHT to attachment sites on the prostate membrane.

Nettle extracts also inhibit enzymes such as 5-alpha reductase that cause testosterone to convert to DHT. It is the DHT metabolite of testosterone that is known to cause benign prostate enlargement, excess facial hair, and hair loss at the top of the head.

Muira Puama

French scientists have identified an herbal extract that has shown libido-enhancing effects in two human clinical studies. Muira puama comes from the stems and roots of the Ptychopetalum olacoides plant and is widely used in the Amazon region of South America as an aphrodisiac, tonic, and cure for rheumatism and muscle paralysis.

Muira puama has been the subject of two published clinical studies conducted by Dr. Jacques Waynberg, an eminent medical sexologist and author of 10 books on the subject. The first study, conducted at the Institute of Sexology in Paris under Waynberg's supervision, was reported in the November 1994 issue of the American Journal of Natural Medicine. The study population consisted of 262 men complaining of lack of sexual desire or inability to attain or maintain erection. After 2 weeks, 62% of patients with loss of libido rated the treatment as having a dynamic effect, while 52% of patients with erectile dysfunction rated the treatment as beneficial. The article goes on to compare muira puama favorably to yohimbine, stating, "Muira puama may provide better results than yohimbine without side effects."

Dr. Waynberg's second study, entitled "Male Sexual Asthenia," focused on sexual difficulties associated with asthenia, a deficiency state characterized by fatigue, loss of strength, or debility, all symptoms of a testosterone deficiency. The study population consisted of 100 men over 18 years of age who complained of impotence or loss of libido or both. A total of 94 men completed the study and were evaluated. Muira puama treatment led to significantly increased frequency of intercourse for 66% of couples. Of the 46 men who complained of loss of desire, 70% reported intensification of libido. The stability of erection during intercourse was restored in 55% of patients and 66% of men reported a reduction in fatigue. Other beneficial effects included improvement in sleep and morning erections.

Treatment with muira puama was much more effective in cases with the least psychosomatic involvement. Of the 26 men diagnosed with common sexual asthenia without noticeable sign of psychosomatic disorder, the treatment was effective for asthenia in 100% of cases, for

120

lack of libido in 85% of cases, and for inability of coital erection in 90% of cases.

The latter finding confirms the broad tonic action of muira puama on conditions of fatigue and stress-related sexual dysfunction. Since muira puama is not an artificial stimulant, it fortifies the system over a period of time. Some men report increased vitality within 2 weeks, while the full effects build over several weeks.

Dr. Waynberg notes that his toxicology studies and observations corroborate the conclusions of the scientific literature on the absence of toxicity of muira puama, which is well tolerated by men in general good health.

One of the earliest scientific studies of muira puama was conducted by another French doctor, Dr. Rebourgeon. His research found the plant to be effective in "gastrointestinal and circulatory asthenia as well as impotence." Three of the most respected scientific authorities on medical herbalism recommend muira puama. In published books, James Duke, Ph.D., chief of the United States Department of Agriculture's Medical Plant Laboratory, and Michael Murray, M.D. recommend muira puama for erectile dysfunction or lack of libido. In addition, Daniel Mowrey, Ph.D., in Herbal Tonic Therapies, stated: "Based on the clinical reports documenting the libido and energy enhancing effects of muira puama, it is possible that this herb induces these positive changes by favorably altering the hormone balance in aging men, i.e., increases free testosterone and/or suppresses excess estrogen".

HUMAN HORMONE MODULATION STUDIES USING NUTRIENTS

In order to ascertain the safety and efficacy of nutrients that are purported to modulate male hormone levels, The Life Extension Foundation sponsored clinical studies to assess the effects of specific supplements on blood levels of testosterone, estrogen, and SHBG. The nutrients tested included various combinations of chrysin, nettle root, maca, ginger root, muira puama, and zinc, along with piperine to enhance the absorption of the chrysin.

The results from the first pilot study showed that nine out of 10 men experienced a significant reduction in serum estradiol (estrogen) levels after only 30 days, compared to baseline. In this brief study, total testosterone increased in seven out of 10 men, but free testosterone increased in only four of the 10 men studied. Other blood parameters were not statistically altered.

A more comprehensive study incorporating a different combination of nutrients resulted in eight out of eight men experiencing increases in free testosterone while levels of the undesirable SHBG declined in seven out of eight men, compared to baseline. Estrogen and other blood parameters were not significantly altered in this study.

A third study was undertaken to evaluate still another combination of nutrients. It revealed that after 30 days, 12 out of 17 men experienced an increase in total testosterone and 11 out of 17 showed an increase in free testosterone, compared to baseline. Again, other blood parameters were not significantly altered.

Based on the results of these studies, a formula called Super MiraForte was developed that contains the combination of chrysin, nettle root, muira puama, piperine, and other nutrients that showed the most potent effects in boosting free testosterone and suppressing estrogen in aging men. For those who would prefer to avoid testosterone-boosting and estrogen-suppressing drugs, 4 capsules a day of Super MiraForte may be considered.

Mandatory Testing

When embarking on a hormone modulation program, medical testing is critical. First, a baseline blood PSA must be taken to rule out existing prostate cancer. Then free testosterone and estradiol tests are needed to make sure that too much testosterone is not being converted into estradiol (estrogen). If estrogen levels are too high, the use of aromatase inhibitors can keep testosterone from converting (aromatizing) into estrogen in the body. Follow-up testing for testosterone, estrogen, and

PSA are needed to rule out occult prostate cancer and to fine-tune your program. It is possible that testosterone patches and creams can increase testosterone levels too much. In that case, blood or saliva testing could save you money by allowing you to use less of the testosterone drug.

There are now natural dietary supplements in development that boost free testosterone levels and suppress excess estrogen. Even when these supplements become available, PSA testing is still mandatory because any substance that increases testosterone should be avoided by most prostate cancer patients.

TESTOSTERONE CAVEATS

Please, after reading all of this, do not just "treat a number." In dealing with sexual function and libido, there is always a large psychological component to enhancing or regaining performance. There are also many physical causes of dysfunction. Do not assume that a certain test number means guaranteed results or you may end up with performance anxiety over that. If you have genuine symptoms, definitely try this protocol; it is well thought out and proven. But remember to include all the other stressors and factors in your life-style into the equation.

CORROBORATING STUDIES

Because of the highly controversial nature of this article, Life Extension has taken the unprecedented step of publishing more than 180 pages of scientific abstracts on our website that are numerically matched to the statements made in this article. This may be the first time for such a massive undertaking, and it reflects the urgent need to convey this information to skeptical physicians so that they will prescribe testosterone and aromatase-inhibiting drugs to individuals whose blood tests indicate a need for these therapies.

PUBLISHED STUDIES

Studies Indicating Testosterone *Does Not* Cause Prostate Cancer

Study 1

"This nested case-control study was based on the cohort of men who donated blood to the Janus serum bank at Oslo University Hospital between 1973 and 1994. Cancer incidence was ascertained through linkage with the Norwegian Cancer Registry. The study included sera from 59 men who developed prostate cancer subsequent to blood donation and 180 men who were free of any diagnosed cancer in 1994 and were of similar age and had similar blood storage time. Neither testosterone, DHT, nor the ratio of testosterone to DHT was associated with risk of developing prostate cancer. These results showed no association, positive or negative, between androgens measured in serum and the subsequent risk of developing prostate cancer" (Vatten et al. Cancer Epidemiology Biomarkers Prev. 1997 Nov; 6: 967. Study conducted at Department of Community Medicine and General Practice, University Medical Center,

Trondheim, Norway [lars.vatten@medisin.ntnu.no]).

Study 2

"We conducted a nested case-control study in a cohort of 6860 Japanese-American men examined from 1971 to 1975. At the time of examination, a single blood specimen was obtained, and the serum was frozen. After a surveillance period of more than 20 years, 141 tissue-confirmed incident cases of prostate cancer were identified, and their stored sera and those of 141 matched controls were assayed for total testosterone, free testosterone, dihydrotestosterone, 3-alpha-androstanediol glucuronide, androsterone glucuronide, and androstenedione. The findings of this study indicate that none of these androgens is strongly associated with prostate cancer risk" (Nomura et al. Cancer Epidemiol. Biomarkers Prev. 1996 Aug; 5: 621-5. Study conducted at Japan-Hawaii Cancer Study at the Kuakini Medical Center in Honolulu, HI 96817).

Study 3

"Prostate cancer was identified in 14% (11/77) of the entire group and in ten men (29%) aged 60 years or older. The median age for men with cancer was 64 years. No significant differences were noted between the cancer and benign groups with regard to PSA level, PSA density, prostate volume, total testosterone level, or free testosterone level. A high prevalence of biopsy-detectable prostate cancer was identified in men with low total or free testosterone levels despite normal PSA levels and results of digital rectal examination. These data suggest that (1) digital rectal examination and PSA levels are insensitive indicators of prostate cancer in men with low total or free testosterone levels, and (2) PSA levels may be altered by naturally occurring reductions in serum androgen levels" (213) (Morgentaler et al. J. Am. Med. Assoc. 1996 Dec 18; 276(23): 1904-6. Study conducted at Division of Urology at the Beth Israel Hospital, Harvard Medical School in Boston, MA 02215).

Study 4

"We conducted a prospective nested case-control study to evaluate the relationships of serum androgens and estrogens to prostate cancer using serum collected at baseline for the Alpha-Tocopherol, Beta-Carotene Cancer Prevention Study. None of the individual androgens or estrogens was significantly related to prostate cancer. These results do not support a strong relationship of serum androgens and estrogens with prostate cancer in smokers" (189) (Dorgan et al. Cancer Epidemiol. Biomarkers Prev. 1998 Dec; 7: 1069-74. Study conducted at Division of Cancer Epidemiology and Genetics, National Cancer Institute, Bethesda, MD 20892-7374 [jd7g@nih.gov]).

Study 5

"We report a nested case-control study of serum bio-markers of 5-alpha-reductase activity and the incidence of prostate cancer. From a cohort of more than 125,000 members of the Kaiser Permanente Medical Care Program who underwent multiphasic health examinations during 1964-1971, we selected 106 incident prostate cancer cases. A control was pair matched to each case on age, date of serum sampling, and clinic location. The adjusted odds ratios and 95% confidence intervals for a one quartile score increase were 1.00 for total testosterone (1.00 = no increased risk), 1.14 for free testosterone, 1.13 for androsterone glucuronide, and 1.16 for 3-alpha-diol G" (Guess et al. Cancer Epidemiology Biomarkers Prev. 1997 Jan; 6: 21-4. Study conducted at Department of Epidemiology, School of Public Health, University of North Carolina, Chapel Hill, NC 27599-7400).

Study 6

"Serum samples were obtained from 6860 men during their study examination from 1971-1975. After a surveillance period of about 14 years, 98 incident cases of prostate cancer were identified. Their stored sera and that of 98 matched controls from the study population were tested for the following: testosterone, dihydrotestosterone, estrone, estradiol, and sex hormone globulin. There was a suggestion that serum dihydrotestosterone levels were lower and the testosterone/dihydrotestosterone ratios were higher in the prostate cancer cases compared with their controls. However, none of these associations or that of the other hormones was strongly significant" (Nomura et al. Cancer Res. 1988 Jun 15; 48: 3515-7. Study conducted at Japan-Hawaii Cancer Study, Kuakini Medical Center, Honolulu, HI 96817).

Study 7

"A case-control study of prostatic cancer was carried out to examine the association between selected physical characteristics and factors related to sexual development and behavior and the risk for this disease. The levels of testosterone (T), dihydrotestosterone, salivary testosterone and T/SHBG (sex hormone binding globulin) did not vary with age. Older men had higher estradiol (estrogen) levels. Further, little association between hormone levels and risk factors was found, except for married subjects having increased serum androgens and heavy subjects having decreased serum androgens (not significant)" (192) (Hayes et al. Eur. J. Cancer Prev. 1992 Apr; : 239-45. Study conducted at Department of Urology, Erasmus University, Rotterdam, the Netherlands).

Study 8

"A population-based nested case-control study was conducted to determine the relation of prediagnostic serum levels of testosterone, dihydrotestosterone, prolactin, follicle-stimulating hormone, luteinizing hormone, estrone, and estradiol to the risk of subsequent prostate cancer. Serum specimens of study subjects were available from a blood collection campaign in Washington County, Maryland, in 1974. There were no significant differences in levels of these hormones between cases and controls, although elevated levels of luteinizing hormone and of testosterone/dihydrotestosterone ratios were associated with mild increased risks of prostate cancer" (194) (Hsing et al. Cancer Epidemiol. Biomarkers Prev. 1993 Jan-Feb; 2(1): 27-32. Study conducted at National Cancer Institute, Division of Cancer Etiology, Bethesda, MD 20892).

Study 9

"The possible relationship between changes in peripheral hormone levels and the occurrence of prostatic pathology was studied in a case-control study involving estimation of various plasma hormones in 368 Dutch and 258 Japanese men, who were grouped as controls and patients with benign prostatic hyperplasia, focal prostatic carcinoma, or clinically evident prostatic carcinoma. There were no significant differences in plasma androgen levels between Japanese or Dutch prostate cancer cases and their respective control subgroups. These findings do not support a correlation between the lower plasma testosterone levels and a lower incidence of prostate cancer in the Japanese men. Furthermore, no significant differences were found between salivary levels of testosterone or the ratio between testosterone and SHBG in the various Dutch subgroups. In Japanese benign prostatic hyperplasia patients, the testosterone to SHBG ratio was significantly increased. In conclusion, the results of this retrospective, cross-sectional study do not indicate that hormonal levels play a primary role in the origin or promotion of prostatic abnormalities" (195) (de Jong et al. Cancer Res. 1991 Jul 1; 51(13): 3445-50. Study conducted at Department of Endocrinology and Reproduction, Erasmus University, Rotterdam, the Netherlands).

Study 10

"Frozen serum samples were analysed for PSA, DHT, testosterone and SHBG, and compared to the diagnosis and tumor stage, grade, and ploidy. DHT levels were slightly lower in patients with prostate cancer but the difference was not statistically significant. There was a trend towards lower DHT values in more advanced tumors. Testosterone levels were lower in patients with cancer than in the control group, but the differences were not significant. There was no correlation between testosterone levels, tumor stage, and ploidy. The testosterone/DHT ratio tended to be higher in patients with more advanced tumors. SHBG levels were lower in patients with cancer than in controls, but the differences were not statistically significant. There were no systematic variations of tumor stage, grade, and ploidy. Within a group, DHT levels tended to be lower among cases and in those with more advanced tumors. No systematic variation was found in the levels of testosterone or SHBG" (197) (Gustafsson et al. Br. J. Urol. 1996 Mar; 77(3): 433-40. Study conducted at Department of Urology, Karolinska Institute at Stockholm Soder Hospital, Sweden).

Study 11

"Index cases and their brothers and sons had a significantly lower mean plasma testosterone content than controls of comparable age. Preliminary data suggest that the metabolic clearance rate of testosterone and the conversion ratio of testosterone to estradiol are relatively high in probands. The observations indicate that familial factors are potent risk factors for the development of prostatic cancer. They also suggest that plasma androgen values in families with prostatic cancer cluster in the lower range of normal and that plasma sex-steroid content is more similar in each brother with or without prostatic cancer than among non-brothers" (198) (Meikle et al. Prostate 1985; 6(2): 121-8).

Study 12

"Baseline sex hormone levels were measured in 1008 men ages 40-79 years who had been followed for 14 years. There were 31 incident cases of prostatic cancer and 26 identified from death certificates with unknown dates of diagnosis. In this study, total testosterone, estrone, estradiol, and sex hormone-binding globulin were not related to prostate cancer, but plasma androstenedione showed a positive dose-response gradient" (199) (Barrett-Connor et al. Cancer Res. 1990 Jan 1; 50(1): 169-73. Study conducted at Department of Community and Family Medicine, University of California, San Diego, La Jolla, CA 92093).

Study 13

"The hypothesis that serum concentrations of pituitary hormones, sex steroid hormones, or sex hormone-binding globulin (SHBG) affect the occurrence of prostatic cancer was tested in a consecutive sample of 93 patients with newly diagnosed, untreated cancer and in 98 population controls of similar ages without the disease. Remarkably close agreement was found for mean values of total testosterone (15.8 in

127

cases and 16.0 in controls), and free testosterone (0.295 and 0.293, respectively), with corresponding odds ratios for the highest vs. lowest tertile of 1.0 (1.00 = no increased risk) for testosterone and 1.2 for free testosterone. Similar close agreement between cases and controls was found for serum concentrations of estradiol, androstenedione, and SHBG, although the mean estradiol level was not significantly lower among cases" (200) (Andersson et al. Br. J. Cancer 1993 Jul; 68(1): 97-102. Study conducted at Department of Urology, Orebro Medical Center Hospital, Sweden).

Study 14

"Modest depression of serum testosterone and estradiol was noted for prostate cancer patients compared to clinic controls, although the differences were not statistically significant. This depression was interpreted to be a likely result of the malignant process rather than a cause of it" (202) (Hulka et al. Prostate 1987; 11(2): 171-82. Study conducted at Department of Epidemiology, School of Public Health, University of North Carolina at Chapel Hill, NC 27514).

Study 15

"The prostate cancer patients had a slightly lower mean free testosterone and mean estradiol/free T ratio than the BPH patients. The mean estradiol/free testosterone ratio was significantly higher in the BPH patients and in the PC patients than in the young controls. It seems possible that the observed age-dependent significant increase in plasma estrogen concentration in the BPH patients may act as a protective factor against prostatic cancer" (203) (Rannik-ko et al. Prostate 1983; 4(3): 223-29).

Study 16

"A fourfold higher relative risk for the development of prostatic cancer was observed for brothers of prostatic cancer cases compared to their brothers-in-law and males in the general population of the state of Utah. Probands and their brothers, and sons of the patients with the disease, had significantly lower plasma testosterone levels than controls of comparable age. This is the first documentation indicating that familial (possibly genetic) factors are potent risk factors for predisposing men to the development of prostatic cancer and in regulating the plasma content of androgens. Our results indicate that plasma androgen levels in families with prostatic cancer are clustered in the lower range of the normal population. They also suggest that plasma androgen content is more similar within each family with cancer than among families without cancer" (204) (Meikle et al. J. Clin. Endocrinol. Metabol. 1982 Jun; 54(6): 1104-1108).

Study 17

"Pretreatment hormone levels were determined in 222 patients with prostatic cancer and their prognostic value assessed. The patients were grouped into yearly survival categories and only those whose cause of death was due to the disease were included in the study. Low concentrations of testosterone in plasma at the time of diagnosis related to a poor prognosis. Patients who died within 1 year of diagnosis had the lowest mean plasma levels of this steroid. The pretreatment mean plasma testosterone concentrations were found to be higher as the survival period of the various groups lengthened. The indications from this study are that poor testicular function is associated with early death from prostatic carcinoma and that the measurement of blood levels of testosterone at diagnosis could provide a prognosis of subsequent life span" (205) (Harper et al. Eur. J. Cancer Clin. Oncol. 1984 Apr; 20(4): 477-82).

Study 18

"Pretreatment plasma concentrations of total testosterone, prolactin, and total estradiol were measured in 123 prostatic cancer patients who were categorized into groups according to the UICC classification. The mean follow-up time was 48 months. Higher pretreatment estradiol and testosterone levels were associated with better survival" (207) (Haapiainen et al. Scand. J. Urol. Nephrol. Suppl. 1988; 110: 137-43. Study conducted at Second Department of Surgery, Helsinki University Central Hospital, Finland).

Study 19

"This cross-sectional study was undertaken to determine whether serum hormones (free testosterone, androstenedione, luteinizing hormone, or prolactin) have any influence on serum prostate specific antigen (PSA) levels in patients with stage A-C prostate cancer. None of the hormones in any of the analyses showed any association to serum PSA values. Serum free testosterone, androstenedione, and luteinizing hormone appeared to have no influence on serum PSA values in nonmetastatic cancer patients" (208) (Vijayakumar et al. J. Natl. Med. Assoc. 1995 Nov; 87(11): 813-19. Study conducted at Department of Radiation Oncology, Michael Reese Hospital, Center for Radiation Therapy, University of Chicago).

Study 20

"Serum levels of testosterone, DHT, androsterone, 5 alpha-androstane-3 alpha, 17-beta-diol (5 alpha-diol), and estradiol were measured by radioimmunoassay in the sera of 9 patients with untreated prostatic cancer and in 11 with benign prostatic hypertrophy (BPH). Although no specific changes in steroid hormone levels in either disease group were found, response patterns of serum T, DHT, and E2 were shown to be those characteristic of male senescence, suggesting a relative predominance of estrogens over androgens" (211) (Isurugi et al. Prostate Suppl. 1981; 1: 19-26).

Study 21

"We studied the effect of exogenous testosterone administration on the serum levels of PSA (prostate-specific antigen) and PSMA (prostate-specific membrane antigen) in hypogonadal men. Serial serum PSA, serum PSMA, and serum total testosterone levels were obtained at intervals of every 2-4 weeks in ten hypogonadal men undergoing treatment with exogenous testosterone, delivered as testosterone enanthate injection or by testosterone patch. A two-tailed, paired t-test failed to demonstrate a significant correlation between serum PSA or PSMA and serum testosterone levels. This study suggests that in hypogonadal men, neither PSMA nor PSA expression is testosterone-dependent" (185) (Douglas et al. J. Surg. Oncol. 1995 Aug; 59(4): 246-50. Study conducted at Department of Surgery, Walter Reed Army Medical Center, Washington, D.C. 20307-5001).

Study 22

"Blood samples were collected from 52 incident cases of histologically confirmed prostate cancer and 52 age- and town of residence-matched healthy controls in Athens, Greece. DHT was associated inversely, significantly, and strongly with the risk of prostate cancer, whereas testosterone was associated marginally positively, and E2 was associated non-significantly inversely with the disease" (Signorello et al. Cancer Causes Control 1997 Jul; 8(4): 632-36. Study conducted at Department of Epidemiology and Harvard Center for Cancer Prevention, Harvard School of Public Health, Boston, MA 02115).

Studies Indicating that Testosterone Causes Prostate Cancer

Study 1

"We conducted a prospective, nested case-control study to investigate whether plasma hormone and sex hormone-binding globulin (SHBG) levels in healthy men were related to the subsequent development of prostate cancer. No clear associations were found between the unadjusted levels of individual hormones or SHBG and the risk of prostate cancer. However, a strong correlation was observed between the levels of testosterone and SHBG (r = 0.55), and weaker correlations were detected between the levels of testosterone and the levels of both estradiol (r = 0.28) and DHT (r = 0.32) (all P < 0.001). When hormone and SHBG levels were adjusted simultaneously, a strong trend of increasing prostate cancer risk was observed with increasing levels of plasma testosterone (ORs by quartile = 1.00, 1.41, 1.98, and 2.60 [95% CI = 1.34-5.02]; P for trend = .004), an inverse trend in risk was seen with increasing levels of SHBG (ORs by quartile = 1.00, 0.93, 0.61, and 0.46 [95% CI = 0.24-0.89]; P for trend = 0.01), and a nonlinear inverse association was found with increasing levels of estradiol (ORs by quartile = 1.00, 0.53, 0.40, and 0.56 [95% CI = 0.32-0.98]; P for trend = 0.03). No associations were detected between the levels of DHT or prolactin and prostate cancer risk. High levels of circulating testosterone and low levels of SHBG--both within normal endogenous ranges--are associated with increased risks of prostate cancer. Low levels of circulating estradiol may represent an additional risk factor" (214) (Gann et al. J. Natl. Cancer Inst. 1996 Aug 21; 88: 1118-26. Study conducted at Department of Medicine, Brigham, and Women's Hospital, Harvard Medical School, Boston, MA).

Study 2

"Basal serum concentrations of sex steroids, sex hormone-binding globulin (SHBG), and gonadotrophins, and the basal levels and response to adrenocorticotropic hormone (ACTH) of adrenocortical steroids, were measured before treatment in 72 patients with prostate cancer and in 42 age-matched healthy controls. Patients aged <60 years with prostate cancer had significantly elevated levels of total testosterone and unconjugated (E1) and total (tE1) oestrone, while patients aged > or = 60 years had significantly elevated levels of total and non-SHBG-bound testosterone (NST), 17-alpha-hydroxyprogesterone and tE1. Gonadotrophins, SHBG levels and relationships between total testosterone and SHBG were normal in both age groups of patients, as were basal levels and ACTH-induced increments of adrenocortical steroids. The patients had normal age-related variations in SHBG and NST and in basal levels and ACTH-induced increments of adrenocortical steroids. There was a significant age-related increase in serum E1 in the control subjects but not in the patients. Patients with metastatic disease had significantly lower E1 levels than had patients without metastases. The results suggest an increased sensitivity of the testes to gonadotrophic stimulation, as well as an increased peripheral oestrogen synthesis in patients with prostate cancer, the latter being most pronounced in younger subjects. Men developing prostate cancer may have been exposed to a combination of elevated endogenous oestrogen and androgen levels for a long time. These findings support the theory of a synergism between oestrogens and androgens as an important factor in the aetiology of prostate cancer" (Carlstrom et al. Br. J. Urol. 1997 Mar; 79(3): 427-31. Study conducted at Department of Obstetrics and Gynaecology, Karolinska Institute, Huddinge University Hospital, Sweden).

Study 3

"A blinded, case-control study was undertaken to determine if hair patterning is associated with risk of prostate cancer, as well as specific hormonal profiles. The study accrued 315 male subjects who were stratified with regard to age, race, and case-control status (159 prostate cancer cases/156 controls). Free testosterone was greater among cases than in controls (16.4 +/-6.1 vs. 14.9 +/-4.8 picogram/mL, $P = 0.02$). Conversely, DHT-related ratios were greater among controls. Data suggest that increased levels of free testosterone may be a risk factor for prostatic carcinoma" (Demark-Wahnefried et al. J. Androl. 1997 Sep-Oct; 18(5): 495-500. Study conducted at Division of Urology, Duke University Medical Center, Durham, NC 27710).

Study 4

"We present the case of a hypogonadal patient in whom a 20-fold increase in prostate-specific antigen and a palpable prostatic nodule developed 6 months into the administration of intramuscular testosterone" (Curran et al. Urology 1999 Feb; 53: 423-4. Study conducted at Department of Urology, Lahey Clinic Medical Center, Burlington, MA 01805).

Study 5

"The metabolic clearance and production rates of testosterone were significantly higher in (prostate cancer) patients than in controls. These results indicate that men with prostatic cancer have elevated clearance and production rates of testosterone without an alteration of estradiol production or clearance" (Meikle et al. J. Steroid Biochem. 1989 Jul; 33(1): 19-24. Study conducted at Department of Internal Medicine, University of Utah School of Medicine, Salt Lake City, UT 84132).

SUMMARY

Before beginning testosterone replacement, comprehensive blood testing is necessary to determine liver-kidney function, and levels of glucose, minerals, lipids, thyroid, free and total testosterone, estadiol, DHT, DHEA, PSA, homocysteine, LH (optional), and SHBG (optional). These tests may be done at your doctor's office or they can be performed directly at a laboratory in your area. A digital rectal exam is also recommended to eliminate the possibility of prostate cancer. Natural testosterone is highly recommended over synthetic types. Nutritional supplements may be added to the diet depending upon test results that can prevent testosterone from cascading into estrogen and DHT.

The following supplements are recommended:

1. Super MiraForte containing chrysin, piperine, nettle, and muira puma boosts free testosterone and suppresses estrogen by acting as a mild aromatase inhibitor, 4 capsules daily.

2. Saw Palmetto/Nettle Formula helps to inhibit SHGB and reduce the effects of excess estrogen, 2 capsules daily.

3. Indole-3-carbinol (IC3) helps neutralize dangerous estrogen metabolites (16-hydroxyestrone), 200-400 mg daily.

4. Zinc functions as an aromatase inhibitor in some men, 80-90 mg daily.

For more information:

The best source for actual case histories of men who successfully used hormone modulation is Dr. Eugene Shippen's book entitled The Testosterone Syndrome. Dr. Shippen provides many interesting details too numerous to be covered in this concise protocol. Another book, Maximize Your Vitality & Potency, by Dr. Jonathan Wright, also contains historical and more technical data about the benefits of testosterone that are, again, too numerous to include in this protocol. These two books are available from the Life Extension Foundation.

Disclaimer

This information (and any accompanying printed material) is not intended to replace the attention or advice of a physician or other health care professional. Anyone who wishes to embark on any dietary, drug, exercise, or other lifestyle change intended to prevent or treat a specific disease or condition should first consult with and seek clearance from a qualified health care professional.

This protocol raises many issues that are subject to change as new data emerge. None of our suggested treatment regimens can guarantee a cure for these diseases.

Much of this information was derived from LE Magazine June 2003

Female Hormone Modulation Therapy

If you are younger than 40 years old, you need not read farther.

By Melissa L. Block, M.Ed.

Hormone deficiencies can wreak havoc with a woman's health and feeling of well-being.

Mainstream medicine has focused on the drop of estrogen as being the culprit behind menopausal miseries. The scientific literature, however, reveals that an imbalance of several hormones is responsible for many of the discomforts and lethal diseases that women face during most phases of their lives.

Concern about the life-threatening side effects of synthetic drugs has caused many women to be deprived of the benefits of safe natural hormone therapy. When hormones are properly replaced, the risk of contracting degenerative disease is reduced. Attaining optimal hormone balance can also dramatically improve women's emotional and physical spheres of life.

This article introduces a new concept to explain why so many females suffer hormone-related problems and provides a simple solution that has been overlooked by most conventional doctors.

With female life span currently hovering around 80 years, the fact is most women spend a significant percentage of their lives in a state of hormone imbalance that began with the onset of menopause. In the U.S. alone, approximately 36 million women have entered menopause, and many of those women experienced troublesome symptoms both before and during "the change."

It's clear that as long as there has been menopause, there have been women who suffer greatly as a consequence of this transition. Once they've passed through this complex transition, women find themselves at increased risk of heart disease, osteoporosis and cancer.

Efforts to help those women who suffer from menopausal symptoms and diseases of aging have moved along two paths. Mainstream medicine's path has led to the widespread prescription of conjugated estrogens, most commonly sold today as Premarin, and synthetic progestins. The second path has led to the development and use of natural estrogens and progesterone. While the first path has led to temporary relief for many women, it has done so at great cost. The second path, although given little credence by the medical mainstream, works without the side effects characteristic of conjugated estrogens and progestins, because its goal is to duplicate the hormonal balance that naturally occurs in a healthy young woman's body.

Conventional vs. natural hormone replacement therapies

The primary aim of both types of hormone replacement therapy (HRT) is to relieve menopausal symptoms. Both have proven capable of achieving this end. HRT research has also focused on its ability to reduce risks of age-related diseases such as heart disease, osteoporosis and cancer.

Possible Premenopause Symptoms

- *Weight gain
- *Bloating
- *Depression
- *Migraine headaches
- *Fibrocystic breasts
- *Breast tenderness
- *Hypothyroidism
- *Uterine fibroids
- *Decreased libido
- *Extremely heavy or extremely painful periods
- *Moderate to severe PMS
- *Endometriosis
- *Infertility
- *Repeated miscarriage

Conjugated estrogens and progestins effectively relieve menopausal symptoms but at the risk of significant side effects, including breast tenderness, vaginal bleeding and mood changes. Some studies have appeared to support HRT's effectiveness at preventing heart disease, but the overall weight of the research data does not support it as preventive medicine against cardiovascular diseases.

The most recent large-scale study showed that this combination of synthetic hormones increased the likelihood of strokes (41%), invasive breast cancer (26%) and heart attacks (29%) in women who used it for less than five years. The results of this study, which involved over 16,000 menopausal women, were so alarming that it was halted prematurely.

Natural estrogens and progesterone, on the other hand, pose little to no risk of adverse effects when they are used properly. Unlike the synthetic progestins and conjugated estrogens, their molecular structure is identical to the hormones made in the human body. When the molecular structure of a hormone is "tweaked" to make it patentable (thus enabling drug companies to charge what they like without fear of competition), it does not function the same as its natural counterpart. This can lead to other actions in the body resulting in unpleasant or dangerous side effects. Natural progesterone and estrogens, which are made from soy or wild yams, are **bioidentical** - indistinguishable from the real thing, both under a microscope and within the human body.

Bioidentical progesterone and estrogens, when used appropriately, also relieve vasomotor symptoms and help to build bone. They pose no increased risk of heart attack, and their physiological effects on the circulatory system are likely to aid in the prevention of cardiovascular disease. Evidence exists that natural (bioidentical) progesterone is more effective at building bone than synthetic estrogens.

Natural hormones are also useful for maintaining or reviving libido during "the change." Unlike any type of synthetic HRT, natural hormones - more specifically, natural progesterone - appear to help prevent breast cancer. An added advantage of natural hormone therapy is that it can be used by women who have yet to pass into menopause. Growing numbers of women in Wester-nized nations begin to experience premenopause symptoms as early as their 30s and 40s (see a partial list of premenopause symptoms, above).

Premenopause symptoms

Most women who experience pre-menopausal symptoms are not ovulating with each menstrual cycle, and so do not make the progesterone needed to balance out the estrogens that build up the uterine lining. Studies have shown that by the age of 35, approximately 50% of women are having at least some anovulatory cycles.

Constant exposure to estrogen-mimicking chemicals in the environment - found abundantly in everything from plastics to cleaning solutions - further elevates these women's estrogen load. The result is an imbalance that hormone expert and author John Lee, M.D. has named estrogen dominance. Estrogen dominance occurs when the tissue-building properties of estrogen are not adequately countered by the normalizing, balancing effects of progesterone, a hormone that can be physiologically supplemented in a manner that mimics the hormonal cycles of a healthy young woman.

A common age for the initial detection of breast cancer is five or more years before menopause. This indicates that factors in play before the menopausal transition - most likely, estrogen dominance - create an ideal environment for the development of breast tumors. According to Dr. Lee and biochemist David Zava, Ph.D., the authors (along with medical writer Virginia Hopkins) of What Your Doctor May Not Tell You About Breast

Cancer (Warner Books, 2002) balancing hormone levels through the proper use of natural progesterone can prevent breast cancer in estrogen dominant women.

Even younger women, including those in their teens and 20s, can suffer from estrogen dominance. Their symptoms may include PMS, weight gain, fibrocystic breasts, bloating, troublesome periods, infertility, endometriosis, depression or repeated miscarriage. Natural progesterone works to relieve symptoms in these younger women as well.

Some menopausal women find that their symptoms are relieved with natural progesterone alone. This is due to two factors: first, estrogens are made in fat cells, which means that heavier (or extremely estrogen dominant) pre-menopausal women may actually continue to be estrogen dominant well into menopause; and second, natural progesterone supplementation has the effect of "waking up" estrogen receptors, increasing their uptake of available estrogens.

Hazards of Oral Contraceptives

Birth control pills contain the same synthetic hormones that have been linked to serious health risks when used after menopause. They have been found to increase risk of cardiovascular disease (strokes, heart attacks and blood clots that can become lodged in leg vessels or vessels that feed the lungs), as well of the risk of developing cancer of the breast, cervix and liver.

The cardiovascular risks of the Pill use are often underestimated. It's likely that the increasing use of oral contraceptives for the symptoms of premenopause will lead to more cardiovascular adverse events, because women in the pre-menopausal age bracket already have elevated risk of such problems.

In some women, oral contraceptives cause depression, anxiety and mood swings. These side effects can be severe enough to affect quality of life and the ability to have healthy relationships.

The use of estrogen drugs in women with premenopause symptoms is not helpful. That's because the last thing any estrogen dominant woman needs is more estrogen, and synthetic progestins can't replace the real thing. Many women with premenopause symptoms end up using oral con-traceptives to control them, and these drugs have their own hazards. This is no surprise when one considers that they contain the same kinds of synthetic hormones found in conventional HRT.

Dr. Lee and other experts have found that natural progesterone is the best treatment for the symptoms of estrogen dominance, and thousands of women have discovered this firsthand.

If natural hormones are superior to synthetic ones, one might ask, where is the research to support this claim? Natural substances cannot be patented, and so the potential for huge profits from their manufacture and sale can't match those of synthetic versions. Because of this fact, it has been impossible to secure the funding necessary for the large-scale trials that could pit natural hormone therapy against the synthetics.

Some studies have been done to show the bioavailability and overall value of natural HRT, but natural hormone researchers have not been able to compete with the enormous, pharmaceutical company-funded studies that have been published on conventional HRT. As a result, most women have been led to believe that conventional hormone replacement therapy was their only option at menopause. The role of synthetic progestins in HRT has been relegated to little more than a preventive measure against uterine cancer. Mainstream medicine has ignored the many important roles natural progesterone plays in reproductive health and in the complete health picture of women in every stage of their life spans.

Natural progesterone, delivered to the body via a skin cream that contains this hormone, is all that many women need to regain and maintain hormone balance. Women who are in or past menopause may also need other hormones, including natural estrogens, testosterone and DHEA.

The many uses of natural progesterone

Progesterone's best-known role is in maintaining a healthy pregnancy. When a woman ovulates, the follicle that has burst to release the ovum becomes the corpus luteum. The corpus luteum secretes anywhere from 4 mg to 28 mg of progesterone per day during the two weeks between ovulation and menstruation, with the average being 22 mg to 25 mg. If pregnancy takes place, the corpus luteum continues to make progesterone throughout the first trimester, playing an indispensable role in maintaining the pregnancy until the placenta can take over the job of providing progesterone. By the third trimester, if ovulation does not occur, no progesterone is made. Ano-vulatory cycles are not easily detected, since menstruation still happens on schedule as long as estrogen does its part. The resulting imbalance of estrogen (which reaches its highest levels at around the 12th day of the menstrual cycle, with the first day falling on the first day of menstruation) and progesterone leads to a condition of estrogen dominance. When this cycle repeats itself frequently, and when it is amplified by environmental estrogens and those made in excess body fat, the body is in a near-constant state of estrogen overload. Estrogen-sensitive tissues get the message to grow and proliferate. By adding progesterone back into each cycle, and gently augmenting progesterone production during ovulatory cycles, balance can be reestablished.

Women who are in or past menopause can also benefit from natural progesterone supplementation. Natural progesterone stimulates the formation of new bone and may help to prevent breast cancer. It counteracts the blood clotting effects of estrogens, improves vascular tone (the ability of blood vessels to stretch and contract in response to the body's requirements), and is believed to protect against the buildup of atherosclerotic plaques and coronary artery spasms that lead to heart attack. It's a gentle mood enhancer and helps to maintain normal libido.

Low thyroid activity is a common problem for postmenopausal women. Estrogen inhibits thyroid hormone activity. Balancing excess estrogens with progesterone enables the body to better utilize thyroid hormone, and can help women to wean themselves off of thyroid hormone replacement drugs.

Progesterone builds bones

One of the main arguments in favor of HRT is that it has been shown in multiple studies to preserve bone mass and protect against osteoporotic fractures. The truth is that while estrogens - even the horse-derived estrogens that comprise Premarin - do preserve bone mass, the overall risks of HRT have been found to outweigh any beneficial effects it might have on bone health.

The synthetic progestin medroxyprogesterone has been found to increase bone density when given to young women who are not menstruating or ovulating. The work of John Lee, M.D., and other like-minded clinicians has shown that natural progesterone has the same bone-building effect in both pre- and postmenopausal women, without the side effects that often occur with the synthetic progestins.

Estrogen maintains bone mass by subduing the activity of osteoclasts - specialized bone cells that break down old bone to make room for new. Progesterone builds bone by stimulating the activity of osteoblasts, bone cells that pull calcium, magnesium and phosphorus from the blood so that it can be incorporated into the bones.

Progesterone and breast cancer

Progesterone modulates much more than the course of a pregnancy. It interacts with estrogen in dozens of ways; the best detailed explanation of these effects can be found in Dr. Lee's writings. The short story on progesterone's relationship with cancer is that while estrogen encourages cellular growth (which is why it is carcinogenic in excess), progesterone encourages cells to differentiate, or mature. Immature cells are more likely to turn into cancerous cells.

Progesterone also encourages cells to undergo apoptosis - programmed cell death. A cell that becomes cancerous avoids apoptosis; it can continue to divide and survive as long as it has fuel and a place to grow. The mechanisms by which estrogen encourages cell growth are also thought to help switch off the genetic machinery that brings on programmed cell death.

Progesterone also reduces the production of a carcinogenic form of estrogen (4-hydroxyestrone) and enhances the production of estriol, a safer, non-carcinogenic estrogen. Breast cancer surgery or biopsy performed during the luteal phase of the menstrual cycle - the phase during which progesterone levels peak - is associated with significant improvements in prognosis and survival time. Progesterone counteracts estrogen's effects on breast duct cells, which are usually the place where breast tumors begin to form.

Estrogen encourages breast duct cell proliferation; progesterone encourages those cells to mature and differentiate. This is how estrogen and progesterone interact during pregnancy to ready the breasts for lactation. Mature, differentiated cells are far less vulnerable to cancerous changes, a fact that explains why women who have had full-term pregnancies are at less risk of developing breast cancer.

How to Supplement with natural progesterone

When taken orally, natural progesterone is almost completely degraded by the liver before it can reach the tissues that need it. Even micronized natural progesterone - now available as a prescription drug called Prometrium® - must be given in high doses to make it through the first pass through the liver. This puts undue stress on the liver and may create metabolites that have harmful effects.

Natural progesterone can be given in the form of suppositories and injections. Both work to move progesterone into the bloodstream, but the first is messy and the latter is inconvenient. The simplest way to supplement with progesterone is transdermally, in the form of a skin cream that contains bioidentical progesterone made from soy or wild yams. When the cream is smoothed onto the skin, the progesterone molecules are absorbed into the layer of subcutaneous fat. The bioavailability of transdermal progesterone has been proven in several studies.

Once absorbed through the skin, the progesterone molecules gradually diffuse into the circulation. This method provides the closest possible approximation to the natural production of progesterone by the ovaries - as long as the dosages are properly timed.

Massage progesterone cream into the breasts, chest, underarms, face, abdomen, buttocks or inner thighs. Rotate the site where cream is applied so that subcutaneous fat cells don't become saturated in any one site. Use a cream that contains 500 mg to 700 mg of progesterone per ounce.

Pre-menopausal women: Women who have not gone through menopause and have estrogen dominance symptoms (including fibrocystic breasts and ovarian cysts) should use 1/4 to 1/2 tsp of progesterone cream, an amount which should provide 20 mg to 40 mg of progesterone, starting on the 8th day of the cycle. (Day one is the first day of menstruation.)

Continue to apply the cream until day 26 of the cycle, and allow seven days (whether menstruation occurs or not) before beginning to apply it again.

PMS: Begin to apply 1/4 tsp of cream on the 12th day after the first day of menstruation and continue until day 26.

Endometriosis: Women with endometriosis should use 1/2 tsp twice a day from days 6 through 26 of the menstrual cycle.

Menopausal and postmenopausal women: Women who are past menopause or who have had a hysterectomy should use 1/4 to 1/2 tsp of cream twice a day for 25 days, followed by five days off. Repeat this cycle for three months, then decrease the dosage to 1/4 tsp twice a day. If you have a uterus and are using supplemental estrogen of any kind, use progesterone cream every day of the month.

Osteoporosis: To help prevent osteoporosis in postmenopausal women, use 1/8 to 1/4 tsp daily from the 12th day to the last day of each monthly cycle. If still menstruating, use the first day of your period to mark the first day of the cycle. Women who have been diagnosed with osteoporosis should apply 1/2 teaspoon morning and night until the first jar is used up, and then 1/4 teaspoon morning and night until the second jar is used up. The latter dosage can be used for maintenance, or can be cut in half once again if bone scans show improvement. In addition to progesterone, supplementation with at least 1000 mg a day of calcium along with magnesium, zinc, boron, manganese, vitamin D and vitamin K are essential in the prevention of osteoporosis.

Progesterone supplementation

Natural progesterone cream is increasingly being used in lieu of synthetic progestin drugs. Like any hormone - natural or synthetic - it's bound to have more significant effects in some people than in others, because of subtle biochemical differences. Fortunately, there is no risk involved in trying it as long as it is used properly. Natural progesterone is now available in an enhanced delivery skin cream (QuSome® encapsulated) to better maintain a consistent youthful level of progesterone in the body.

Disclaimer

This information (and any accompanying printed material) is not intended to replace the attention or advice of a physician or other health care professional. Anyone who wishes to embark on any dietary, drug, exercise, or other lifestyle change intended to prevent or treat a specific disease or condition should first consult with and seek clearance from a qualified health care professional.

This protocol raises many issues that are subject to change as new data emerge. None of our suggested treatment regimens can guarantee a cure for these diseases.

Changes in body composition during post-menopausal hormone therapy: a 2 year prospective study.

Arabi A, Garnero P, Porcher R, Pelissier C, Benhamou CL, Roux C

BACKGROUND: Post-menopausal hormone therapy (pHT) induces changes in both body composition and bone mineral density (BMD). METHODS: In 109 post-menopausal women beginning either tibolone 2.5 mg (n=29), tibolone 1.25 mg (n=42) or estradiol 2 mg plus norethisterone acetate 1 mg (E2 + NETA) (n=38), we assessed body composition, total and regional BMD by dual energy X-ray absorptiometry, and the serum bone alkaline phosphatase (BAP), osteocalcin and the urinary excretion to type I collagen C-telopeptide (CTX) at baseline and after 2 years. RESULTS: At baseline, BMD at all sites correlated negatively with age and years since menopause, and positively with lean mass and fat mass (r=0.42, P<0.001 and r=0.26, P=0.006 at the total femur). During treatment, BMD increased at all sites (P<0.001), and serum BAP, osteocalcin, and urinary CTX decreased in all groups (P<0.001). Lean mass increased whereas android fat and android obesity index decreased. The increase in BMD at all sites correlated positively with changes of lean mass at 2 years. CONCLUSIONS: Both fat mass and lean mass are related to BMD in post-menopausal women, the relationship being strongest with lean mass; an increase in lean mass and a change in distribution of body fat are observed during treatment with E2 + NETA and tibolone.

Hormone Modulation in your Community

There are many clinics, physicians, OBGYN's who specialize in hormone modulation therapy around the country. However, this being a new science, there may not be one in your area.

The third largest compounding pharmacy in the country is College Pharmacy. They are located in Colorado Springs, Colorado. They compound prescriptions for physicians all over the country and mail the product directly to the patient. If you contact them, they may be able to refer you to a physician in your area.

College Pharmacy
Phone: (800) 888-9358
(719) 262-0022
3505 Austin Bluffs Parkway, Suite 101
Colorado Springs, CO 80918
info@collegepharmacy.com

Call Clinix and they may have a referral in your area. If not, they can arrange for you to obtain the proper blood work in your community. The results are then faxed directly to Clinix. At that point, they can help you with only one office visit, and periodic follow-up blood test.

Clinix
Work:303-721-9984
Fax:303-267-4566
7030 South Yosemite
Centennial, CO 80112

144

Understanding the Reference Ranges

When physicians review a patient's blood test results, their only concern is when a particular result is outside the normal laboratory "reference range." The problem is that standard reference ranges usually represent "average" populations, rather than what the optimal range should be to maintain good health.

The lethal consequences of faulty reference ranges have been discussed for many years in Life Extension magazine. As more studies show that a person's health can be severely impaired when physicians rely on standard reference ranges, it becomes imperative for you to educate yourself about "optimal" ranges to avoid becoming a victim of medical ignorance.

It now appears that most standard reference ranges are too broad to adequately detect health problems or prescribe appropriate therapies on an individual basis.

An example of flawed reference ranges can be seen in blood tests used to assess thyroid status. A long-standing controversy has been how to best diagnose thyroid deficiency. Conventional doctors rely on thyroid blood tests, whereas alternative physicians also look for other signs and symptoms of thyroid deficiency. A recent article in The Lancet reveals surprising new findings about reference ranges that may shake up current theories about assessing individual thyroid status.

Before discussing The Lancet article, the reader should be acquainted with the serious consequences of a thyroid hormone deficiency. Aging people encounter a variety of ailments that doctors often attribute to problems other than thyroid deficit. Some of the most noticeable symptoms caused by low thyroid are poor concentration, memory disturbances, cold hands and feet, accumulation of excess body fat, difficulty in losing weight, menstrual problems, dry skin, thin hair and low energy. Some specific disorders related to thyroid deficiency include depression, elevated cholesterol, migraine headaches, hypertension and infertility.

Broda O. Barnes, M.D., Ph.D. was a physician-scientist who dedicated more than 50 years of his life to researching, teaching and treating thyroid and related endocrine dysfunctions. In his book entitled, Hypothyroidism: The Unsuspected Illness, Dr. Barnes described over 47 symptoms that may be related to poor thyroid function. During his many years of research and practice, Dr. Barnes condemned conventional doctors who ignored obvious clinical manifestations of thyroid deficiency.

According to Dr. Barnes:

"The development and use of thyroid function blood tests left many patients with clinical symptoms of hypothyroidism undiagnosed and untreated."

In lieu of blood tests, Dr. Barnes advocated that patients measure their temperature upon awakening. If the temperature is consistently below normal ranges, this is indicative of a thyroid deficiency. The box below provides specific instructions on how best to measure your body temperature in order to assess your thyroid hormone status.

Dr. Broda Barnes believed that 40% of the adult population suffers from thyroid deficiency. Based on the percentage of adults now taking prescription drugs to treat depression, elevated cholesterol, high blood pressure and other conditions, Dr. Barnes' observations about the epidemic of thyroid deficiency may now be validated.

What's wrong with thyroid blood tests?

The Lancet is one of the most prestigious scientific journals in the world. It often reports new medical findings that defy conventional wisdom. According to an article published in the August 3, 2002 issue of The Lancet, the problem with thyroid blood tests may be faulty "Reference Ranges" that fail to reflect what the optimal level of thyroid hormone should be in a particular individual.

Thyroid Self Testing

Upon awakening before you get out of bed, put a thermometer under your arm with no clothing between the bulb and your armpit. Leave it there for 10 minutes (use snooze alarm if you wake up to an alarm clock). Just drowse for that time lying still. If the armpit method is too inconvenient, you can put the thermometer in your mouth for three minutes (or until the electronic thermometer registers a temperature).

After the appropriate number of minutes take the thermometer out and read it, writing down the result right away. This is known as your Early AM Basal Temperature, and the "normal" should be between 97.8 and 98.2. The reading taken by armpit is somewhat lower and somewhat more accurate than by mouth. If you have a low-grade infection your temperature may read higher than your "normal." If it is within the range mentioned above, you should repeat the procedure every other day for two weeks. If you are a menstruating female, do it on the 2nd and 3rd day of your period.

If your average temperature over a two-week period is lower than 97.8 to 98.2, you are probably hypothyroid. If it is higher, then you are probably hyperthyroid (or you have an infection somewhere).

As stated earlier in this article, standard laboratory reference ranges represent "average" populations, rather than what the optimal range should be. Back in the 1960s, for instance, the upper reference range for cholesterol extended to 300 (mg/dL). This number was based on a statistical calculation indicating that it was "normal" to have total cholesterol levels as high as 300. At that time, it was also "normal" for men to suffer fatal heart attacks at relatively young ages. As greater knowledge accumulated about the risk of heart attack and high cholesterol, the upper limit reference range gradually dropped to the point where it is now 200 (mg/dL).

The same situation occurred with homocysteine reference ranges. Up until recently, it was considered normal to have a homocysteine blood reading as high as 15 (mm/L). Most reference ranges now provide a chart showing that homocysteine levels above 7 increase risk of heart attack and stroke.

It's not just blood laboratory reference ranges that fail to provide physicians and patients with optimal numbers. For example, when your blood pressure is checked, a diastolic number up to 90 (mm Hg) is considered normal. Yet a diastolic blood pressure reading over 85 is associated with an increased stroke risk. A high percentage of people over age 60 have diastolic readings over 85 and this is the age group most vulnerable to stroke. So when your doctor checks your blood pressure and says it's normal, your response should be that "normal" is not good enough, since it is also normal for people over age 60 to suffer a stroke. Instead, you should ask your doctor what is the "optimal" range. In the case of diastolic blood pressure, taking steps to keep it at 85 or below could greatly reduce long-term vascular damage. It is important to note that mid-life hypertension predisposes people to stroke later in life, so keeping blood pressure readings in optimal ranges is important at any age.

Scientists are now examining thyroid hormone reference ranges and their findings indicate that it may be time to change the way laboratories report TSH results.

The Thyroid Stimulating Hormone (TSH) Test

The standard blood test used to determine thyroid gland hormone output is the thyroid stimulating hormone test (TSH). When there is a deficiency in thyroid hormone, the pituitary gland releases more TSH to signal the thyroid gland to produce more hormones.

When the TSH test is in "normal range," doctors usually assume that the thyroid is secreting enough thyroid hormone. The question raised by The Lancet authors, however, is whether today's reference range for TSH reflects optimal thyroid hormone status.

The TSH reference range used by many laboratories is between 0.2 to 5.5 (mU/L). A greater TSH number is indicative of a thyroid hormone deficiency. That is because the pituitary is over-producing TSH based on lack of thyroid hormones in the blood. Any reading over 5.5 alerts a doctor to a thyroid gland problem and that thyroid hormone therapy may be warranted.

The trouble is that the TSH reference range is so broad that most doctors will interpret a TSH reading as low as 0.2 to be as normal as a 5.5 reading. The difference between 0.2 and 5.5, however, is an astounding 27-fold. It would seem almost absurd to think that a person could be in an optimal state of thyroid health anywhere along this 27-fold parameter, i.e. TSH readings between 0.2 and 5.5.

A review of published findings about TSH levels reveals that readings over 2.0 may be indicative of adverse health problems relating to insufficient thyroid hormone output. One study showed that individuals with TSH values over 2.0 have an increased risk of developing overt hypothyroid disease over the next 20 years. 15 Other studies show that TSH values over 1.9 indicate abnormal pathologies of the thyroid, specifically autoimmune attacks on the thyroid gland itself that can result in significant impairment.

More ominous is a study showing that TSH values over 4.0 increases the prevalence of heart disease, after correction of other known risk factors. Another study showed that administration of thyroid hormone lowered cholesterol in patients with TSH ranges of 2.0 to 4.0, but had no effect in lowering cholesterol in patients whose TSH range was between 0.2 and 1.9. This study indicates that in people with elevated cholesterol, TSH values over 1.9 could indicate that a thyroid deficiency is the culprit causing excess production of cholesterol, whereas TSH levels below 2.0 would indicate no deficiency in thyroid hormone status.

Doctors routinely prescribe cholesterol-lowering drugs to patients without properly evaluating their thyroid status. Based on the evidence presented to date, it might make sense for doctors to first attempt to correct a thyroid deficiency (based on a TSH value over 1.9) instead of first resorting to cholesterol-lowering drugs.

In a study to evaluate psychological well being, impairment was found in patients with thyroid abnormalities who were none-the-less within "normal" TSH reference ranges.

Defying the reference ranges

The authors of The Lancet study stated that, "the emerging epidemiological data begin to suggest that TSH concentrations above 2.0 (mU/L) may be associated with adverse effects."

The authors prepared a chart based on previously published studies that provide guidance when interpreting the results from TSH blood tests. Here are three highlights from their chart that may be useful in determining what your TSH values really mean:

- TSH greater than 2.0 Increased 20-year risk of hypothyroidism and increased risk of thyroid autoimmunity[15]
- TSH greater than 4.0 Greater risk of heart disease
- TSH between 2.0 and 4.0 Cholesterol levels decline in response to thyroxin (T4) therapy

Despite presenting these intriguing findings, The Lancet authors stated that more studies are needed to define optimal TSH level as between 0.2 and 2.0 instead of between 0.2 and 5.5. As a health conscious person, however, this type of precise information provides an opportunity to correct a medical condition that has been unresponsive to mainstream therapies, or possibly prevent disorders from developing in the first place.

This means if you suffer from depression, heart disease, high cholesterol, chronic fatigue, poor mental performance or any of the many other symptoms associated with thyroid deficiency, you may want to ask your doctor to "defy the reference ranges" and try thyroid replacement therapies.

Measuring thyroid hormone levels

TSH is just one blood test that doctors use to assess thyroid status. Other blood tests measure the actual amount of thyroid hormone found in the blood.

The primary hormone secreted by the thyroid gland is called thyroxin (T4). The T4 is then converted in the peripheral tissues into metabolically active triiodothyronine (T3).

Doctors often test for TSH and T4 together, but this may not accurately reflect thyroid deficiency in tissues throughout the body. One study found that psychological well being could be improved if T3 (like the drug Cytomel) is added to T4 (like the drug Synthroid) therapy, while maintaining thyroid function broadly within the standard reference ranges. What this means is that even when TSH and T4 blood tests are within normal ranges, a person can still be deficient in peripheral T3 and benefit from Cytomel therapy.

Since T3 is the metabolically active form of thyroid hormone, some doctors use it exclusively in lieu of T4 drugs like Synthroid. The FDA's recent notice to ban synthetic T4 drugs like Synthroid because of inconsistent potencies helps to validate the following statement made by Dr. Broda Barnes more than 50 years ago:

"Patients taking thyroid replacement therapy have much better improvement of symptoms with natural desiccated thyroid hormone rather than synthetic thyroid hormones."

While the FDA has found many problems with T4 drugs, the T3 drug Cytomel has produced consistent clinical results and is not a subject of the FDA's proposed ban. Dr. Barnes fought the drug companies over synthetic T4 drugs for years and recommended desiccated thyroid (Armour) as the therapy of choice for most patients.

An article in the New England Journal of Medicine described a study in which patients with hypothyroidism showed greater improvements in mood and brain function if they received treatment with Armour thyroid rather than Synthroid (thyroxin). The authors also detected biochemical evidence that thyroid hormone action was greater after treatment with Armour thyroid.

All hormone reference ranges may be antiquated

It's not just thyroid hormone deficiency that goes unrecognized by so many physicians. Conventional medicine has neglected virtually all the hormone imbalances that develop as a part of growing older. The result is that aging people suffer a variety of discomforts and lethal diseases that are correctable and preventable if simple hormone adjustments are made.

150

Standard versus Optimal

A person's risk of contracting lethal disease, suffering debilitating disorders and prematurely aging can be partially predicted based on the findings of blood tests that assess hormone levels. What follows are the Standard Reference Ranges compared to the Optimal Ranges for a 60-year old male:

Hormone Standard Reference Range Optimal Range

Test	Normal	Optimal	Units
DHEA	42-290	280-500	ug/DL
Insulin (fasting)	6-7	Under 5	uU/ml
Free Testosterone	6.6-18.1	15-22	pg/mL
Estradiol	0-54	10-30	pg/mL
TSH	0.2-5.5	Under 2.1	mU/L

Aging men, for instance, often suffer from excess production of insulin and estrogen, with simultaneous deficiencies of free testosterone and DHEA. If a physician were to test blood levels of all four of these hormones, the standard "reference ranges" are so wide that most men would fall into the so-called "normal" category.

Standard reference ranges indicate that dangerously high insulin and estrogen levels are "normal" in elderly men. So are heart attacks, stroke, cancer, benign prostate enlargement, weight gain, Type II diabetes, kidney impairment and a host of other diseases that are associated with excess insulin and estrogen.

For instance, the standard reference ranges for free testosterone and DHEA show that very low levels are perfectly "normal" for aging men. It's no coincidence that these same aging men (with low testosterone/DHEA) suffer high rates of depression, memory loss, atherosclerosis, senility, impotency, high cholesterol, abdominal obesity, fatigue and a host of other diseases related to low blood levels of testosterone and DHEA.

When it comes to assessing hormone status, standard reference ranges have failed aging humans in a terrible way. The reason is that reference ranges are adjusted to reflect a person's age. Since it is normal for an aging person to have imbalances of critical hormones, standard laboratory reference ranges are not flagging dangerously high levels of estrogen and insulin or deficient levels of testosterone, thyroid and DHEA. The box "Standard versus Optimal" on this page shows standard hormone blood reference ranges for men and compares them to what the "optimal" ranges should be.

Most doctors still believe that imbalances of life-sustaining hormones are "normal" for aging people. These physicians think that nothing should be done to restore hormone profiles to youthful ranges (and almost never test hormone levels anyway).

The problem is that aging people no longer accept that they should contract the diseases that happen to fit into their age category. In other words, more 65-year olds are demanding the health and vitality enjoyed by a younger person. This is not possible if 65-year olds allow their hormone levels to stagnate in today's archaic reference ranges. If you are 80 years old and are told that your hormone profile is normal for your age, tell your doctor that you would prefer the hormone profile of a 25-year old since you perceive a 25-year old as having more vitality and a reduced risk of contracting lethal diseases than an 80-year old.

Aging people who adjust their hormone profiles to fit a more youthful profile can turn back some of the effects that time has inflicted on their bodies. In order to accomplish this, however, you must defy the standard laboratory reference ranges and seek the blood values of a much younger person.

ARTICLE II.   VITAMINS & MINERALS

It has long been known that vitamins and minerals are essential nutrients for the human body. But you may wonder what these nutrients do for the body, how much is enough and how much is too much. The following information should help answer these questions. It tells what various vitamins and minerals do for the body, in what foods they are found and what the Recommended Dietary Allowances and potential overdose risks are for each.

Taking an overdose means giving the body vitamins and minerals in a quantity greater than is necessary. Excess of a particular vitamin or mineral can pose risks as serious to health as a deficiency of that nutrient. Nutrients are interrelated and an excess of one nutrient can upset the balance the body requires of other nutrients. A variety of healthful foods eaten in moderation will likely supply the body with the nutrients it needs. Usually a vitamin/mineral supplement is not necessary.

The Recommended Dietary Allowances (RDA) can provide guidance in determining the amounts of nutrients needed by the body. The RDAs are the amounts of nutrients essential to meet the known nutritional needs of nearly all healthy persons in America. The RDAs given in this publication are for adult men and women ages 25 to 50.

Abbreviations

   mg = milligrams
   ug = micrograms
   m = male
   f = female
   RE = retinal equivalents (1 RE = 5 IU; IU = International Units)
   TE = alpha tocopherol equivalents

Minerals	RDA	Function	Major sources
1. Calcium	800 mg	Assists in clotting of blood and building of bones and teeth. Promotes proper functioning of nerves, heart and muscle.	All forms of milk, cheese (except cottage cheese and cream cheese) and ice cream.
2. Iodine	150 ug	Promotes proper functioning of thyroid gland.	Seafood, iodized salt.

3. Iron	10 mg(m) 15 mg(f)	Makes hemoglobin, the red substance in blood. Transports oxygen to and from cells.	Organ meats, oysters, lean meats, eggs, leafy green vegetables, dried peas and beans, enriched breads and cereals.
4. Magnesium	350 mg(m) 280 mg(f)	Needed for contraction of nerves and muscles and for normal metabo- of potassium and calcium. Activates many- enzyme systems, involved in carbohydrate metabolism and protein synthesis.	Nuts, whole grains, dried peas and beans, milk, green leafy vegetables.
5. Phosphorus	800 mg	With calcium, helps build bones and teeth, aids in release of energy from carbohydrates, fat and protein; aids in formation of genetic material and cell membranes.	Meat, poultry, fish, eggs, dried peas and beans, milk and milk products.
6. Zinc	15 mg(m) 12 mg(f)	Constituent of many enzymes important in metabolism, aids in wound healing, needed for normal growth, especially during childhood, and for normal taste sensation.	Meat, fish, egg yolk, milk, oysters, whole grains.
7. Selenium	70 mg(m) 55 mg(f)	With vitamin E, helps protect cells from oxidative damage; involved in fat metabolism.	Seafood, kidney, liver, meat, cereals.
8. Vitamin A	1,000 ug RE(m) 800 ug RE(f)	Helps eyes adjust to dim light. Helps keep skin and lining of mouth, nose, throat and digestive tract healthy and resistant to infection.	Liver, butter, cream, whole milk, cheese, egg yolk, dark green leafy vegetables, yellow and orange fruits and vegetables, fortified products.

9. Vitamin D	5 ug	Helps body use calcium and phosphorus to build and maintain strong bones and teeth.	Fortified milk, exposure to sunlight, fatty fish, eggs, liver, and butter.
10. Vitamin E	10 mg TE (m) 8 mg TE (f)	Helps keep red blood cells intact. An antioxidant, protects vitamin A and essential fatty acids from oxidation. Helps maintain normal muscle metabolism.	Vegetable oils, especially wheat germ oil, margarine.
11. Vitamin K	80 mg(m) 65 mg(f)	Involved in synthesis of proteins required for blood clotting	Green leafy vegetables, dairy products, meats, eggs, cereals, fruits.
12. Vitamin C	60 mg	Helps hold body cells together and strengthens walls of blood vessels; helps in healing wounds; helps body to build bones and teeth; aids in the absorption of iron.	Citrus fruits, green peppers, tomatoes, strawberries, cantaloupe, cabbage, broccoli, kale, potatoes.
13. Thiamin (B_1)	1.5 mg(m) 1.1 mg(f)	Helps body cells obtain energy from food. Helps keep nerves in healthy condition. Promotes good appetite and digestion.	Pork, liver and other organs, wheat germ, whole grain or enriched cereals and breads, soybeans, peanuts and other legumes and milk.
14. Riboflavin (B_2)	1.7 mg(m) 1.3 mg(f)	Aids in utilization of protein, fat and carbohydrate for energy. Promotes healthy skin, eyes, clear vision.	Milk, organ meats and enriched breads and cereals.
15. Niacin	19 mg(m) 15 mg(f)	Helps body cells produce energy from food. Helps to maintain health of skin, tongue, digestive tract and nervous system.	Lean meat, fish, poultry, liver, kidney, whole wheat and enriched cereals and breads, peanuts.

16. Folacin	200 ug(m) 180 ug(f)	Needed for normal productions of red and white blood cells, proper development of fetus and infants, maintenance of a healthy adult nervous system, maintains normal functioning of the gastrointestinal tract, and manufacture of basic cell genetics (RNA and DNA).	Liver, yeast, deep green leafy vegetables, avocado, oranges and orange juice, navy, lentil and lima beans.
17. Pyridoxine (B_6)	2.0 mg(m) 1.6 mg(f)	Needed for protein metabolism. Helps to build blood cells.	Meat, liver, kidney, whole grain cereals, peanuts, green leafy vegetables.
18. Cobalamin (B_{12})	2 ug	Needed to build healthy red blood cells. Needed for normal growth in children	Found only in foods of animal origin, like liver, meat, milk, eggs, cheese.

Which MVMS are best?

Under ideal conditions supplements should not be necessary. However, the fact is that our diets have undergone dramatic changes over the past several decades. In fact, seven out of every ten deaths in the United States are now directly related to diet and lifestyle. Excessive fat, sugar, and salt are linked to our biggest killers-heart disease, cancer, and stroke.

Although it has been almost 29 years since this report was written, on can only assume the situation has worsened.

The 1988 Surgeon General's Report on Nutrition and Health acknowledged:

"What we eat may affect our risk for several of the leading causes of death for Americans, notably, the degenerative diseases such as: Atherosclerosis; coronary heart disease; strokes; diabetes; and some types of cancer.

These disorders, together, now account for more than two-thirds of all deaths in the United States." That is quite an acknowledgment for the Surgeon General's office to make. We bring this to your attention because it is our belief that the more you know about this subject, the better you can prepare yourself. The average American family is simply unaware of the health consequences of an improper diet. Primarily because they don't know what a proper diet consists of. You have already learned this in the previous section.

Even if we could achieve the ideal diet and nutrition intake (which is extremely difficult these days), we would still face the challenge of an environment that is much different than several decades ago. Pollution, herbicides, pesticides, and other environmental contaminants place tremendous additional stress on our immune systems and other body systems. Supplementing our diet offers much protection from these new pollution challenges.

Aside from all of the literature on the nutrients an average American needs, you are no longer an average American. You are an athlete. Now, you need more and better nutrition than the "average American".

Your body needs the best it can get to perform at the level that you now require.

Therefore, there is widespread agreement that a daily MVMS (multi-vitamin mineral supplement) is a sensible and inexpensive "insurance" policy for your health and well-being. Experts from Harvard University (both the Medical School and School of Public Health), The Center for Science in the Public Interest (CSPI), and dozens of other highly-respected (and conservative) institutions have long-recommended a well-balanced MVMS. Unfortunately, the important question for most of us has not been, "Should I take a multi?" but, "WHICH multi should I take".

If you're an adult, you're multivitamin choices can get complicated with several subcategories denoting you as a man (pre- or post-40) or a woman (pre-menopausal, postmenopausal or pregnant/prenatal).

After figuring out which category you fit in, your choice of an actual product can be mind-bogglingly difficult for the sheer number of products on the market. Even after answering which category you fall into, you're still faced with dozens of "basic" multivitamins and dozens of "senior" products, and dozens of ultra-super-mega-others. To help simplify your decision-making process, the experts at one of the national companies, whose specific job is to review every multivitamin/mineral supplement on a battery of 10 minor criteria in 5 major is shown below.

They use a mathematically weighted system whereby Science and Safety scores carry more "weight" than other categories. This review process culminates in an Overall Score (0-100 points). This point method allows the comparison to each other. It would be impossible for us to provide detailed, specific information on each product, but we have tried to give you an overall suggestion based on this one companies score.

Below we have listed a few of the MVMS that are rated in the upper 10% and are readily available. Some are available through multi-level marketers, and other are on the shelf of various retail stores. All you need do is do a web search by product name and manufacturer. That will tell you where price and availability.

Suggested MVMS Choices

The following choices are not recommendations. At the time of this printing, they have the following scores from one particular supplement rating company. Some of the products they rated were omitted because I could not determine where they could be purchased.

Name	Manufacturer	Score	Availability	Cost 30 day supply
WOMENS HEALTH				
LifePak Women	Pharmanex	95	Pharmanex	$77
Daily Balance - Dr. Susan Lark	Doctors Preferred	95	drlark.com	$50
LifePak Prenatal	Pharmanex	93	Pharmanex	$50
Dr. Art Ulene's Optimal Vitamin Formula for Women	Feeling Fine Company	92	Retail Outlets	$10
Solgar Female Multiple	Solgar	91.5	Internet	$23
GNC Multiples – Women's VitaPak	GNC	91	GNC	$28
GNC Multiples – Women's Ultra Mega	GNC	87.5	GNC	$15
Women's Nutritional System by Rainbow Light	Rainbow Light	87	Internet	$42
High Energy Pack	Kirkland	88	Costco	$5
Women's Symmetry by Vitanica	Vitanica	87	vitanica.com	$14
Nature Made Women's Pack	Nature Made	85.5	Retail Outlets	$10
Nutirlite XX	Nutrilite		Internet	$75
MENS HEALTH				
Nutriex - Health	Nutriex	96	nutriex.com	$40
Nutriex - Sport	Nutriex	96	nutriex.com	$50
LifePak for Men	Pharmanex	95	Pharmanex	$70
Vitox	Pharmanex	95	Pharmanex	$45
Clinical Nutrients for Men	Phyto Pharmica	94	Internet	$23
Mega Men, Timed Release Tablets	GNC	93	GNC	$12
GNC Multiples - Men	GNC	90.5	GNC	$26
High Energy Pack	Kirkland	88	Costco	$5
Nutirlite XX	Nutrilite		Internet	$75

Anti-Oxidants

What are anti-oxidants and free radicals?

Anti-oxidants fight free radicals. So what are free radicals? Free radicals play an important role, in both health and disease, and have been implicated in countless human disease processes. Free radicals are vital to human health. These molecules (Reactive Oxidant Species) are extremely important to human metabolic processes.

Any molecule can become a free radical by either losing or gaining an electron and molecules containing these uncoupled electrons are very reactive. Once free radicals are initiated, they can propagate by becoming involved in chain reactions with other less reactive types. The resulting chain reaction compounds generally survive longer in the body and therefore increase the potential for cellular damage.

A free radical has three stages: the initiation stage, propagation and finally, termination. They are terminated or neutralized, by nutrient antioxidants, enzymatic mechanisms, or by recombining with each other. The aim is to attain a delicate balance between free radical activity and optimum antioxidant activity, thereby achieving a state of balance (homeostasis).

The three known free radicals are hydroxyl, super oxide and peroxide. If they are not neutralized into "good oxygen", free radicals can speed up the aging process and play a major part in the development of degenerative and/or chronic diseases.

Free-radical damage. Created by normal body functions, free radicals are unstable molecules that can damage cells and cell DNA. Doctors know from autopsy evidence that brain cells are particularly vulnerable. Researchers have tested the effect of a variety of so-called antioxidants-- which neutralize free radicals--with mixed results. A substance called cur cumin (from the herb turmeric) significantly improves brain function in animals with memory deficits, Cole said; so do preparations that include alpha-lipoic acid and vitamins C and E, to name a few.

Vitamins that are anti-oxidants

Vitamins A, C and E are all anti oxidants. Tests imply that 5000mg of vitamin E is an effective daily dose. Vitamin C is a more effective anti oxidant than vitamin E but passes through your system quickly and must be taken frequently throughout the day.

Vitamin C is best taken at least two hours before or after meals and sugared drinks and/or first thing in the morning and last thing at night.

VITAMIN E occurs in food in several forms - alpha, beta, delta, and gamma-tocopherols and alpha, beta, delta and gamma tocotrienols. Most E supplements contain only the alpha tocopherol form because it is believed to have the greatest biological activity. Research at the University of California, Berkeley reported in the Proceedings of the National Academy of Sciences that gamma-tocopherol is able to quench certain free radicals that alpha-tocopherol does not. Of the E vitamins it has been stated that only gamma-tocopherol gets rid of peroxynitrite, a highly destructive nitric oxide radical.

It has been suggested that high levels of alpha-tocopherol in the blood can *reduce* the level of the gamma form. Different tocopherol forms appear to have complementary but not identical functions.

Both alpha and gamma-tocopherol occur in natural Vitamin E, but the vitamin supplements generally sold as vitamin E contain only alpha-tocopherol, which may then displace gamma-tocopherol in the body. Gamma-tocopherol may be a more effective anti-oxidant than alpha-tocopherol. (Christen S., et al., Gamma-tocopherol traps mutagenic electrophiles such as NOx and complements alpha-tocopherol: Physiological implications. Proc. Natl. Acad. Sci. USA, vol 94, pp. 3217-3222, Apr 1997.)

A major new survey of 47 health studies concludes that Vitamin E plays not only an important role in preventing or alleviating neurological disorders, but that natural Vitamin E, as opposed to synthetic products, supplies far more concentration to the brain and other body tissues. Natural Vitamin E puts five times the concentration in the brain than does the synthetic version, the survey said. "The importance of Vitamin E in maintaining neurological structure and function has been well documented in clinical research." summary of scientific studies from 1980 to 1997 concluded: "Long-term Vitamin E deficiency is associated with a progressive neurological syndrome that can be alleviated by Vitamin E therapy."

Comparing natural Vitamin E to synthetic, the survey said: "It appears that the nervous system has a marked preference for natural-source Vitamin E, which may be significant in treatment of neurological disorders. Studies have demonstrated a preference for natural-source Vitamin E by various body tissues, including the brain and spinal cord, compared to synthetic Vitamin E" the survey said. "There was preferential uptake of natural-source Vitamin E by the lung, red blood cells, blood plasma and brain. The brain showed the highest discrimination for natural-source Vitamin E. The concentration of natural source Vitamin E in the brain increased gradually to a five-fold higher concentration than the synthetic isomer after five months, suggesting that natural-source Vitamin E will be significantly more available to the brain than the equivalent intake of synthetic Vitamin E."

The study continued: "Oxidative damage has been implicated in a number of neurological disorders and diseases, and the majority of available research has demonstrated a protective role for Vitamin E ... Research shows that antioxidant therapy has "significantly beneficial effects in reducing associated disability," the survey said.

It has been suggested that vitamin E is best taken in the morning or during the day (never at night) and that it be taken at a different time to other supplements for best results. Avoid taking it with magnesium supplements.

TOCOTRIENOL is a much neglected component of vitamin E. In addition to the four tocopherols, another related series of compounds, tocotrienols, have been discovered which are less widely distributed in nature. While tocopherols are predominantly found in corn, soybean and olive oils, tocotrienols are particularly rich in palm, rice bran and barley oils. Therefore, vitamin E is the term used for eight naturally occurring essential fat-soluble nutrients: alpha, beta, delta & gamma tocopherols plus a class of compounds related to vitamin E called alpha, beta, delta and gamma tocotrienols. Comparatively, the tocotrienol structure differs by possessing three double bonds in their side chain rather than being saturated.

Tocotrienols have been shown to elicit powerful antioxidant, anti-cancer and cholesterol lowering properties. Some studies have confirmed that tocotrienol activity as an antioxidant, anti-cancer and cholesterol reducing substance to be much stronger than tocopherols. Tocotrienols were once thought to be of lesser nutritional value than the tocopherols, it is apparent that their activity and importance rank them as one of the most important class of nutritional compounds for the prevention and treatment of disease.

Please note: Extract from the book written by Lavon J Dunne, "Nutritional Almanac":

"Vitamin E has a tendency to raise blood pressure when it is given in high doses to someone who is not accustomed to it. Therefore initial intake should be small, and as tolerance rises, the dosage should be gradually increased".

Other antioxidants

PYCNOGENOL/OPC Grape seed/Pinebark extract provides a weapon against premature aging of living structures. Oxygen free radicals are believed to be responsible for the deterioration of these structures. The lengthening of life expectancy, observed for 50 years in the western world seems to have reached its limits: little by little we have found remedies for the accessible causes of aging. What remains is oxygen, of which nobody had thought 20 years ago and of which we now know constitutes life's principal wear and tear factor. Oxygen free radicals do have a physiological mission to accomplish: the burning of refuse matter, but we should prevent them destroying the sensitive structures of the living cell. OPC offers protection against oxygen free radicals supposes a long term, even permanent use of the scavenging antidote. Used in therapeutics for 40 years, it has never provoked direct or secondary effects of a toxic nature. This is hardly surprising because we find it in the various foods consumed since the beginning of history. There is extensive information on the Internet about Pycnogenol and check here for information about OPC.

Cur cumin A substance called cur cumin (from the herb turmeric) significantly improves brain function in animals with memory deficits, Cole said; so do preparations that include alpha-lipoic acid and vitamins C and E, to name a few.

Alpha-lipoic acid

Coenzyme Q10 (CoQ10) or ubiquinone is an essential cofactor of the electron transport chain as well as a potent free radical scavenger in lipid and mitochondrial membranes. Because of its strong antioxidant properties, coenzyme Q-10 is being tested in patients with degenerative neurological diseases, Parkinson's disease, Huntington's disease, ALS/MND and multiple sclerosis at major medical centers, including the University of Rochester Medical School and the University of California at San Diego. The hope is that coenzyme Q-10 can slow down progression of the diseases. Andrew Weil, MD personally takes 100 milligrams of coenzyme Q-10 once a day with food as a general health-booster and feels it is harmless. Dr. Weil is a nationally-known physician and director of the Program in Integrative Medicine at the University of Arizona and also a graduate of Harvard College and Harvard Medical School. He has published many books on health and healing. Dr. Weil's website is at : http://www.dr.weil.com/. Many studies suggests that Coenzyme Q10 may be better strategy than vitamin E in treatment of neuro-degenerative diseases in increasing survival time. Oral administration of coenzyme Q10 increases both brain and brain mitochondrial concentrations. The results provide further evidence that coenzyme Q10 can exert neuroprotective effects that might be useful in the treatment of neuro-degenerative diseases.

ASTAXANTHIN is a carotenoid compound usually made from a microalg called Haematococcus pluvialis. Some forms are indissoluble (many anti oxidants are fat or water soluble). As beta carotene (a preliminary stage of vitamin A) is sometimes recommended as an anti oxidant and Astaxanthin supplies carotenoids, it should be safe to take - although a precise dosage has yet to be established.

Astaxanthin has been claimed to be ten times more effective than beta carotene and 100 times more effective than vitamin E in preventing lipid peroxidation. However, as vitamin E and Astaxanthin possibly work in different ways it may be advisable to take both as they could complement each other.

CAROTENOIDS are a group of anti oxidant nutrients found in many fruits and vegetables. They are more easily absorbed in supplement form and even more effective if taken with highly coloured fruits and vegetables such as carrots, tomatoes, watermelon, beets, etc. high in carotenoids. Like all anti oxidants, carotenoids work better in combination than if taken alone. For example, beta-carotene boosts the anti oxidant activity of lycopene (Wahlqvist, et al American Journal of Clinical Nutrition 1994 Vol 60,936-943). Carotenoids include Beta-carotene, Alpha carotene, Cryptoxanthin, Lycopene, Lutein and Zeaxanthin. Each performs a slightly different function at a different level and is dependant on other carotenoids for its effectiveness. Synthetic carotenoids have little biological effect and should be avoided. Ensure you choose naturally derived carotenoids suspended in an oil base

PHENOLICS are naturally occurring anti oxidant substances found in the skins of many fruits, vegetables and herbs. Fruits and vegetables with brightly coloured skins are generally considered to be relatively high in phenolics as are the skins and seeds of the grapes (vitus vinifera) used to make red wine.

Primary anti oxidants:
1. Vitamins A, C and E
2. PYCNOGENOL/OPC Grape seed/Pine bark extract
3. Coenzyme Q-10
4. Carotenoids
5. Phenolics
6. Soy Isoflavonoids

Summary: Ideally we would like to have all of the above listed anti-oxidants and MVMS's at the appropriate designated times where we would attain maximum benefit. However, that being pretty impossible, an excellent MVMS with some or most of the above listed anti-oxidants should suffice for most of us.

Personally from a cost vs. quality perspective, I opt for the Kirkland Brand High Energy Pack from Costco. It is rated 88 out of a possible 100. A 90 day supply consisting of 90 packets only cost $16.00 the last time I purchased it. That is only $5.00 a month. In addition, I take Coenzyme Q-10, and Saw Palmetto. I also put use soy milk in my cereal and in my daily Latte'. I do this to get the benefits of the Soy Isoflavonoids. Keeping in mind, that I eat extremely well, I feel this protocol is very adequate for me. *–Kip*

Personally, I've been taking Nutrilite brand multivitamins (DoubleX in particular) for years and swear by them. Although they aren't cheap, they've always rated very high in independent studies and Nutrilite is one of the largest distributors of vitamins in the world. They've been producing vitamins for over 70 years now. Owning much of their own land and production facilities allows them to maintain higher quality products then the others. To find out more about these supplements visit: www.kellyi.wwdb.biz and enter the access code "health". You can order online from that site at retail or wholesale - if you become an IBO (independent business owner). Otherwise, find a local Quixtar (Nutrilite) distributor to purchase them from. *– Robb*

New on the scene is DNA testing for the purpose of matching your body with the correct vitamins and supplements for optimum health. A customized supplementation pack can be optained that is matched to your specific body. Email Robb at rk@Q45.net if you'd like more information about this.

Chapter Eight

Never Say Diet

If you follow and understand this program, not only will you be in better health and in the best shape of your life, you will know more about nutrition than most of the doctors that you meet.

My goal is to get you thinking about living an active lifestyle, and to minimize the importance of food in your life. Diet is becoming a dirty word among nutrition experts. Not only are diets usually unsuccessful, but over time, repeatedly losing weight and gaining it back, can make long-term weight loss more difficult and may even shorten your life. Studies find, for example, that people with fluctuating weight have a 75% higher risk of dying from heart disease than people with more stable weight, even if it is higher than optimal.

IMPORTANT! When you diet by simply cutting calories (like the Weight Watchers points program), you lose not only fat, but metabolism-revving muscle a well. When you gain weight back, it's mostly fat. If you lose 20 lbs. and gain it back, you are usually worse off than had you never lost the weight in the first place because you probably lost 15 pounds of fat and 5 pounds of lean mass (muscle). Yet, when you gained the 20 pounds back, it is ALL FAT, and you now have less lean mass than you did before you lost the 20 pounds in the first place. As a result, your metabolism is lower, and it will become more difficult to maintain your weight.

So, go forward and design a personalized plan of nutrition and exercise that will maximize your muscularity and minimize your body fat. Become who you really are.